Eat & BEAT DIABETES

WITH PICTURE PERFECT WEIGHT LOSS

Also by Dr. Howard M. Shapiro

Dr. Shapiro's Picture Perfect Weight Loss
Dr. Shapiro's Picture Perfect Weight Loss Shopper's Guide
Dr. Shapiro's Picture Perfect Weight Loss 30-Day Plan
Dr. Shapiro's Picture Perfect Weight Loss Cookbook
Dr. Howard Shapiro's Picture Perfect Prescription

Eat & BEAT DIABETES WITH PICTURE PERFECT WEIGHT LOSS

The Visual Program to **Prevent** and Control Diabetes

Dr. Howard M. Shapiro and Chef Franklin Becker

Photographs by Bill Milne

HARLEQUIN

EAT & BEAT DIABETES WITH PICTURE PERFECT WEIGHT LOSS
ISBN-13: 978-0-373-89218-1
© 2010 by Howard Shapiro and Franklin Becker
Photography © 2010 by Bill Milne

The health advice presented in this book is intended only as an informative resource guide to help you make informed decisions; it is not meant to replace the advice of a physician or to serve as a guide to self-treatment. Always seek competent medical help for any health condition or if there is any question about the appropriateness of a procedure or health recommendation.

Library of Congress Cataloging-in-Publication Data
Shapiro, Howard M., 1943-
    Eat & beat diabetes with picture perfect weight loss : the visual program to prevent and control diabetes /Howard M. Shapiro and Franklin Becker ; photographs by Bill Milne.
      p. cm.
      ISBN 978-0-373-89218-1 (pbk.)
    1. Diabetes—Diet therapy—Popular works. 2. Weight loss—Popular works.
    I. Franklin, Becker. II. Title. III. Title: Eat & beat diabetes with picture perfect weight loss.
    RC662.S53 2010
    616.4'620654—dc22
    2009042995

For Kay von Bergen Shapiro—a woman of exceptional intelligence
and courage who loves to laugh at the craziness of life while reaching out
to others with kindness and compassion. My constant support and
true partner, she doesn't just "make a life for me";
in my mother's words, she makes it wonderful.
—Howard Shapiro

For my children, Sean and Rory Becker, and my wife, Jennifer.
Without all of you, my life would be empty.
—Franklin Becker

ACKNOWLEDGMENTS

It is always a pleasure for authors to acknowledge the people who helped make their books possible and who have been companions along the route of conceiving, writing, editing and assembling the final works.

This book begins with our agent, Carol Mann, who brought us together with one another and with our publisher. In doing so, she also brought us to Donna Hayes, Harlequin publisher and CEO, who has been a consistent champion of our unique approach to fighting diabetes and living a sustainably healthy life.

We are grateful beyond words to our superb editor at Harlequin, Deborah Brody, who shepherded both book and authors gently through the process and offered exquisite understanding during some very difficult extenuating circumstances.

Deborah's assistant, Alex Colon, set a new standard for organization and attention to detail. As point man for all the myriad pieces of the puzzle, he proved to be both a peerless professional and a pleasure to work with.

Also at Harlequin, we express our thanks to publicity genius Shara Alexander, who grasped our message, articulated it beautifully and saw at once how to get the word out; to product manager Amy Jones; to creative director Margie Miller; and to art director Tara Kelly, who created the design for packaging our message and oversaw its implementation brilliantly.

Production of the book was graced by an exceptional team, including the brilliant photographer Bill Milne, a man who is not only a superb professional but who also consistently went the extra mile to make this book just right. Bill was ably assisted by the very talented and gracious Paul O'Hanlon and by office manager Lisa Cichocki, who managed to juggle myriad schedules of myriad people and get all of us where we were supposed to be when we were supposed to be there.

As has been true of all of Dr. Shapiro's books, Diane Vezza served as the food stylist for the many demonstrations that bring our message to life. Diane is sui generis in her work and calm under pressure on the job—no matter what. And kudos to Diane's assistant, Joan Parkin, who did the food preparation that was so essential to the final result.

Phyllis Roxland, Dr. Shapiro's longtime nutritionist, provided her expertise as always and worked tirelessly to make the book a success, while Susanna Margolis, another longtime team member, contributed her editorial skills. Dr. Shapiro would not have been able to devote the time needed to the book *and* run his practice without the support of assistant Alexandra Lotito, the office technology ace, who worked on the book even from her sickbed, while Gerri Pietrangolare, often assisted by Sharon Griffith, kept the office running.

Dr. Shapiro also expresses his thanks to his brother and sister-in-law, Michael and Andee Shapiro, for their support—when it was very much needed—during the writing of this book.

And Chef Franklin extends his gratitude to his parents for their ongoing support and to the sous-chefs and pastry chefs, past and present, who helped him perfect his trade and develop his diabetes-fighting recipes.

We both are grateful to all the chefs around the country who gave their time and effort and created recipes for this book.

CONTENTS

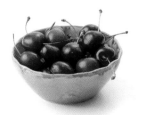

Eat a whole cup of cherries for less than half the calories of 3 licorice sticks. See page 105.

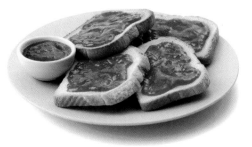

Have 4 slices of light toast with sugar-free jam for just one-third of the calories of a cranberry scone. See page 124.

Look and Lose
Need a great start to your day? See page 123 for your best choice.

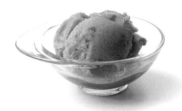

Though better for you than ice cream, a 1-cup scoop of sorbet has just as much sugar. See page 110.

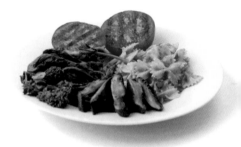

You can eat all of this for practically half the calories of a bowl of pasta and marinara sauce. See pages 68-69.

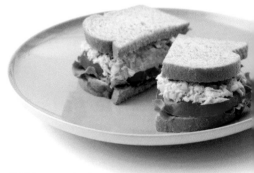

Eat tuna salad on whole wheat for lunch instead of a burger. See page 33.

The Diabetes Danger
and the Team That Will Help You Beat It

Nobody likes to pick up a book, open it to page 1 and get scared out of their wits.

Well, we're not setting out to scare you, but we're here to tell you that there is a danger out there that you and your family need to be aware of.

You need to be aware of it because it has the potential to affect you and everyone you know—your spouse, your friends, your relatives, the people you work with and, above all, your children.

It's the sixth most potent killer of Americans, and 8 percent of us have it right now—including one of the authors of this book.

It's the leading cause of blindness, amputations and kidney failure.

It can triple our risk of heart attack and stroke, and it routinely damages sight, hearing, sleep, mental health and sexual performance.

It is the disease that can eat us alive.

It is diabetes, and it is stealing our health, our well-being, our longevity and our ability to enjoy our lives to the fullest.

Every day, another 2,200 Americans are diagnosed with this disease. It is projected that a third of the population born in 2005 will contract diabetes. It afflicts nearly a quarter of all Americans sixty and older.

If you're a woman who was diagnosed with diabetes before the age of forty, your life span is likely to be shortened by fourteen years. If you're a man, lop off eleven years.

Don't have the disease? Not yet, anyway. For in addition to the 24 million of us diagnosed with diabetes, the Centers for Disease Control and Prevention estimate that some 57 million people are prediabetic—with abnormal blood sugar levels—but don't know it.

Anyone who is obese or even overweight is at risk for the disease. Since our own Department of Health and Human Services says that 64 percent of us—129.6 million Americans—are overweight or obese, that means that most of us are in danger of getting diabetes.

And just when you thought the news couldn't get worse, it does. *Thanks to the stunning increase in childhood obesity, we are seeing a substantial rise in the occurrence of diabetes in young children—as young as eleven and twelve.* In general, in fact, the disease is showing up earlier and earlier. Between 1990 and 2000, for example, while the prevalence of diabetes in adults increased 33 percent overall, it rose a staggering 76 percent among people between the ages of thirty and thirty-nine. Meanwhile, college students and even teenagers are suffering the kind of heart ailments typically reserved for the elderly—thanks to the lowering age of diabetes onset. It means, unfortunately, that all these young people will have more time to accumulate the damage diabetes causes to the blood vessels and nerves—and more time means more damage.

We can sum it all up in this awful truth: diabetes and the excess weight that so often lead to it are a major cause of the reality that today's rising generation is the first ever expected to have a shorter life span than that of its parents.

It's a costly truth, too, and we're all going to pay for it. Today, we shell out an estimated $105 billion per year for the direct and indirect costs of diabetes. That's nothing compared to what we'll be spending to pay for the disastrous, debilitating and doubtless chronic health problems of the future.

If you're diabetic now, you probably already know most of this. You also know you have a tough row to hoe.

A SPECIAL NOTE FROM THE DOCTOR

If your routine blood test shows an abnormal level of sugar, your doctor is likely to order a number of other tests. Three tests in particular are typically used; here's what doctors look for in the tests as possible signals of diabetes.

TEST	LOOKING FOR
Random plasma glucose	Glucose $\geq$ 200 mg/dL
Fasting plasma glucose (tested following a fast)	Glucose $\geq$ 100 mg/dL
Two-hour plasma glucose (tested two hours after ingesting 75 grams of glucose)	Glucose $\geq$ 200 mg/dL

If you think you're free and clear of the disease, think again. Get your blood sugar level checked at your next physical to make sure you're not walking around with a prediabetic condition you just don't know about.

And if you are overweight or obese, it's time to admit the truth to yourself: you're at direct risk of contracting a killer disease.

Did we scare you enough? Well, here's the good news: we know who can control and even cure your diabetes if you're diabetic today, and who can prevent you from ever getting the disease if you're not.

You.

With no other medical condition is the power for cure as clear-cut. With no other medical condition is the responsibility as explicit. It's simple: *you're in charge.* All you have to do is *follow the principles we'll outline in this book.* When you do, *you'll beat diabetes and all its complications—and you'll achieve and maintain a healthy weight loss.* And in this book, we'll tell you how to do it absolutely deliciously.

DIABETES AND YOUR WEIGHT

What is diabetes, and why is weight so central a factor in getting the disease—and therefore so pivotal an issue for controlling or curing it?

In a way, it's all about energy—the energy the body uses for getting out of bed in the morning, running a marathon, doing the work we're paid to do, focusing on our studies, dancing our socks off at a party. As we all remember from high school biology, the digestive process breaks down the food we eat into the various chemical substances our cells need to work properly. One of those substances is glucose, which is basically a sugar, and which just happens to be the body's main energy source. Some of the glucose derived from the digestive process is used right away—say, for getting out of bed and sprinting to work—and some is stored for future use, such as the socks-peeling dancing later tonight.

The regulation of glucose levels—how much gets released into the bloodstream now for the sprint to the office, how much gets held back in storage for the dancing later—is dictated mainly by the gland known as the pancreas, right behind the stomach. The process by which the glucose is controlled is a highly complex interaction of chemicals and hormones, including two hormones—glucagon and insulin—that are manufactured in the pancreas and which work in opposition to each other. Glucagon takes glucose out of storage and sends it into the bloodstream, thus *raising* the level of blood sugar, while insulin moves glucose from the bloodstream into the cells, thus *lowering* the blood sugar level. When everything is working normally, the pancreas produces just enough of both hormones to keep the amount of glucose in the bloodstream perfectly balanced.

If there's not enough insulin, however, the body's cells won't get the message about absorbing glucose. Or there may be enough insulin, but the cells may not be working right; they're suddenly not responding to the insulin message. Either way—whether the insulin is insufficient or ineffective—the glucose gets stuck at the point where it normally enters the body's cells. In other words, the body's ability to regulate its indispensable source of energy, glucose, is disrupted. That's diabetes.

What happens when the glucose can't enter the cells? It builds up in the blood instead, then passes through the kidneys and overflows into the urine. That's why one of the classic symptoms of diabetes is frequent urination, and it's also where diabetes gets its official name, diabetes mellitus—from an ancient Greek verb, *diabainein,* meaning "to pass through," and from a later medieval Latin addition, *mellitus,* meaning "honeyed," indicating the sweetness of glucose passing through the body.

If the disruption to the glucose-regulation mechanism goes untreated, the blood sugar will continue to rise. What can result is a chronic illness comprising a range of health problems and presenting the risk of even worse medical complications. What it means to be a diabetic is that you are constantly working to control these problems and cure the illness.

The complications can be very profound indeed. Hardening of the arteries leading to heart attack and stroke, blood vessel disorders that often lead to kidney failure or blindness, nerve damage, infections that in the worst case can require the amputation of limbs: all the organs of the body are at risk because of the damage diabetes does to the blood flow, and all sorts of disease and debilitation can result.

Until recently, doctors used to talk about "juvenile" and "adult" diabetes. No more. Now, the spread of "adult" diabetes among younger and younger individuals—a direct effect of that rise in childhood obesity—has rendered the two terms imprecise if not obsolete. Instead, medicine speaks of type 1 diabetes, in which the pancreas produces either not enough insulin or none at all, and type 2 diabetes, the type we will focus on in this book, in which the body's cells simply don't respond to the insulin.* We call such cells insulin-resistant, and what makes them insulin-resistant is that the individual is overweight or obese.

That's why there's that special relationship between being overweight and becoming diabetic. Here's how it works.

* Other, less common forms of diabetes include gestational diabetes, which affects from 2 percent to 5 percent of pregnant women and typically resolves spontaneously after childbirth, and certain rare forms of the disease that may derive from genetics, infection, malnutrition and even drugs or surgery.

Once the insulin factory in the pancreas produces insulin, it needs to be captured by the body's cells. For that purpose, each cell has a highly sensitive area that almost literally attracts insulin as it circulates. These areas are called receptors—specifically, insulin-binding cell receptors, because they grab the insulin and bind it with glucose so the glucose can enter the cell and produce energy. As body fat increases, however, the number of those insulin-binding receptors goes down. The sensitivity of the receptors also declines. Bottom line? The insulin receptors stop functioning adequately, the pancreas simply tires out from trying to produce ever bigger amounts of insulin to compensate for the receptors' inadequacy and the body becomes unable to produce enough insulin to maintain a normal blood sugar level.

What this suggests, of course, is that if the person lost weight, the insulin-binding receptors would start functioning again. Then the blood sugar level would return to normal, the health problems would go away and the medical complications might even unwind and conceivably go into reverse.

In fact, that's exactly what happens. And that's the really good news about diabetes today.

Healthy weight loss has long been the first line of attack against the disease of type 2 diabetes. It is the first line of defense in preventing it, and it is the cure for people who already have it. Lose weight, and the symptoms disappear; maintain the weight loss, and the symptoms will not reappear. Regain weight, however, and the disease comes back.

For years, healthy weight loss for diabetes meant avoiding certain foods. Diabetics did not have to give up everything they loved, but their eating was confined: the range of ingredients and styles of cooking was necessarily limited. Today, however, the latest laboratory research provides some very, very good news for diabetics who take care to eat in a way that keeps their disease under control or prevents its occurrence. What the *researchers have found is that there are particular nutrients that actually fight the disease* over the long term. Their names aren't a secret—*fiber, phytonutrients, soy protein*, and the *so-called good fats*: monounsaturated, polyunsaturated, and omega-3 fatty acids—but think of them as secret weapons in the battle against all the complications of diabetes. Clearly, the foods that contain these diabetes-fighting ingredients should be part of every diabetic's eating plan, and we'll show you how in this book—deliciously.

But the best news of all is that the kind of eating that leads to healthy weight loss and the kind of eating that controls diabetes are exactly the same. Here's why. Diabetes is not just a disease; it is also a risk factor. It is a component of what doctors have labeled *metabolic syndrome*—a combination of medical disorders including high blood pressure, high total cholesterol, high LDL cholesterol (the bad cholesterol), low HDL cholesterol (the "good" cholesterol), high triglycerides and overweight or obesity. The more of these components of metabolic syndrome a person has, the greater his or her chances of suffering life-threatening complications. But having even one component puts a person at risk for these complications. The eating principles you'll learn in this book—and the weight loss that can follow—address all the components of metabolic syndrome.

Need to lower your blood pressure? Lose weight healthfully.

Need to curb your LDL cholesterol count? Lose weight healthfully.

Got a potential problem with heart disease? Lose weight healthfully.

Diagnosed as diabetic or prediabetic? Lose weight healthfully.

Want or need to lose weight healthfully?

Create an eating plan that avoids what diabetics should avoid and includes what we now know diabetics should eat. You'll lose weight. Guaranteed. And you'll have created a weight management plan that is a health prescription for everyone—for you, for your family and especially for your children.

That's the eating plan you'll find in this book—informed by a doctor and nutritionist and deliciously prepared by a gourmet chef and his team of colleagues.

YOUR TEAM TO BEAT DIABETES

Medical science can tell us what to eat, but it takes expertise in cuisine to tell us how. We've put the two together and assembled a team that translates all the science about fighting diabetes—including the new secret weapons—into a menu of meals and snacks, drinks and desserts, picnics and parties that are easy to prepare and absolutely superb to the taste. We'll tell you why this eating plan works so well to bring you to the healthy weight that is your best weapon against diabetes and metabolic syndrome, and we'll show you how you can make such a plan an integral part of your life.

And by the way, it's easy to do. The result is not just a battle plan for the disease but a healthy weight-loss plan for every family—the best, simplest, most delicious way there is to ensure a vital, long life.

The core of the team are the coauthors of this book—a gourmet chef who is also a diabetic and a doctor specializing in weight loss.

The chef is Franklin Becker, who was diagnosed as a diabetic at the age of twenty-seven. This graduate of the Culinary Institute of America turned on a dime and transformed his cooking, finding new ways to create dazzling dishes that are healthful and flavorful. In these pages, he'll put to work his own special genius, his experience as chef at such venues as the legendary Brasserie in New York City and the contributions of numerous gourmet-chef colleagues to present a range of dishes, from the simplest and quickest recipe to the highest of haute-cuisine concoctions—all delicious, and all bullets against the disease he lives with and keeps under control.

Chef Franklin is joined by physician and writer Howard Shapiro, author of the bestselling *Picture Perfect Weight Loss* series of books. Dr. Shapiro also has an intimate and tragic association with diabetes, for his sister died of complications from the disease, while his Picture Perfect Weight Loss methodology early on defined the correlation between an eating plan for healthy weight loss and a battle plan against diabetes. From Dr. Shapiro, you'll find out about the stunning new research discoveries that make Chef Franklin's recipes so important, and you'll learn the simple but powerful secrets to preventing or controlling this major killer disease simply by following the principles in this book.

Dr. Shapiro is particularly noted for his Picture Perfect Weight Loss food comparisons, which, in his earlier books, showed readers a range of food options and compared the weight-loss consequences of each. The food comparisons you'll see in this book will assess each food option in terms of not just weight loss but also its specific power to fight diabetes and its complications. Such visual comparisons are among the most powerful tools we can bring you in the fight *against* diabetes and *for* healthy weight loss. They make the healthy option vividly clear—and Chef Franklin's recipes, as well as the recipes of a team of celebrity chefs, then show you how to make the healthy option a gourmet treat.

As both authors want you to know, this is a book for all the family. Not just because being overweight is dangerous and scary, but because achieving and maintaining a healthy weight is so important for everyone's health—and if you're a parent, especially for your children's health. After all, everybody eats. Everybody has to eat. And a healthy weight happens through eating, not through not eating. More about that in the next chapter.

CHAPTER 1

The Secret to Healthy Weight Loss, Diabetic or Not

Do you like chili? Who doesn't? So take a look at the two dishes of chili shown here.

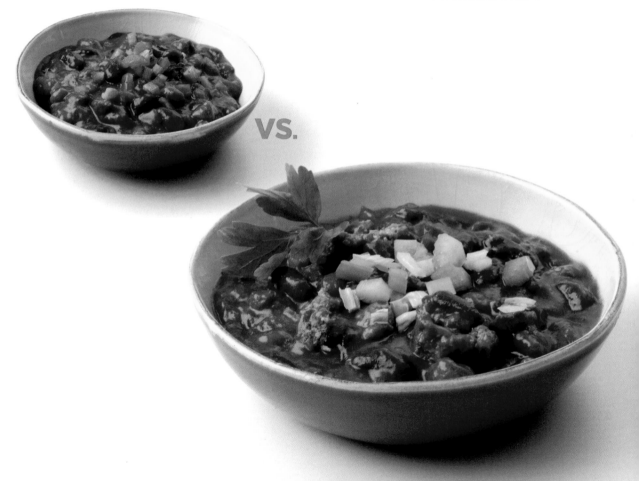

VS.

The one on the left is your standard meat chili. It tastes good—no doubt about it—but at 530 calories, with a heavy dose of saturated fat, it's also the equivalent of a preassembled unit of unhealthy weight gain that, down the road, could contribute to all sorts of unhappy consequences for your body, your well-being and your longevity. In other words, it isn't just that your waistline will increase because of the calorie load; you're also increasing your load of cholesterol and triglycerides and adding to your body's insulin resistance—all thanks to the kind of fat this meat-based dish provides.

You can't taste the veggie-and-bean chili dish pictured on page 1 (see recipe on page 17), but take the word of this book's coauthors, the photographer who took the picture, the photography session stylist and the publisher's representative that it is a major treat for the taste buds. And at 150 calories, a low level of saturated fat and an utter lack of cholesterol, it's also a feel-good food where healthy weight loss is concerned.

But that's only for openers. With its high content of fiber, soy protein and other plant-based nutrients, this chili actually constitutes a weapon of proactive diabetes prevention. It easily earns a **Beat Diabetes award, given to those foods or meals shown to be particularly effective in fighting the disease—not just medically, but because the food or dish has been road tested for taste, convenience and impact on weight loss.** That's also why this chili is such a good bet for any lunch or dinner table—whether you're diabetic or not.

Why are we showing you these photos—the legendary food comparison demonstrations pioneered by Dr. Shapiro? There are two reasons.

First, because they illustrate precisely why the way you eat is a two-edged sword in the ongoing effort we all must wage for health in general and to prevent or control diabetes in particular. One edge plays defense, mitigating the adverse impacts of increased cholesterol and triglycerides (which can lower insulin resistance) and of C-reactive protein (a signal of the kind of inflammation that can portend cardiovascular problems). The other edge—and it's the real secret of this book—plays offense, actually attacking the components of metabolic syndrome and beating back diabetes and its consequences.

The second reason for showing you this demo—and all the others featured in this book—is that the real secret to healthy weight loss is choice. And as has been shown time and again, the best way to understand what that means is to see it for yourself. This book is all about helping you to see—literally, in the case of these food comparisons—the great difference you can make in your life by the way you choose to eat.

We can't say it too often: the tools to beat diabetes are in your hands. The key to healthy weight loss is also in your hands. The two things—beating diabetes by preventing or controlling it and healthy weight loss—are equivalent. The way you choose to eat is the single path to achieving both results. It's as simple as that.

THE BEAT DIABETES PYRAMID: A LOT TO CHOOSE FROM

Choice happens every day, several times a day. Mealtimes, snack times, the coffee break and at the meeting, the nibbles at cocktail hour, the attack of the munchies while watching TV or before bed: all of these situations, plus a zillion more you know only too well, offer us choices about eating.

In fact, unless you head for a restaurant every time you feel hungry, the choosing starts even earlier—at the market, if you're the one who does the shopping for your household, or in the kitchen, if you do the food preparation and cooking.

For people diagnosed as diabetic or prediabetic—or for those told by their doctors that they ought to lose weight—the choices used to be limited. They were told precisely what not to eat and what they could eat. That meant carrying around a list of forbidden foods when they went to the market or out to a restaurant. It meant sitting down to a meal thinking about the foods they were supposed to avoid. On many diets, it meant counting calories, measuring portions, eating only at certain times of day or eating certain combinations of foods, deprivation and often going hungry.

Not anymore. Today we know that there is a bounty of foods playing both defense and offense in the fight to control weight and stay healthy. We know that neither dieting nor deprivation works and that counting and measuring are not just out-of-bounds for today's lifestyles but pointless in terms of controlling weight and enhancing health. We know, in short, that **food is not the enemy of the healthy weight loss that can prevent or control diabetes; it is instead the way to ensure healthy weight loss. It is precisely the way to beat diabetes.**

You've seen "food pyramids" before. They have become the standard mechanism for laying out a particular eating plan—for good reason. Pyramids not only define the kinds of foods the plan advocates but also map the proportionate representation of foods in the plan.

Here's the Beat Diabetes Pyramid. It's the perfect guide to the choices that will help you lose weight healthfully and prevent or control diabetes.

This book devotes a chapter to each level of the pyramid—Chapters 4 through 8—telling you how to apply the pyramid on a practical basis, day by day, in order to achieve healthy weight loss and beat diabetes. But in general, here's what the Beat Diabetes Pyramid demonstrates.

Just as the pyramid is necessarily widest at the base, let vegetables be the foods you eat most—most often, most regularly and most *of.* Raw or cooked, from a can or a package, in soups or stir-fries, vegetables should be the foundation of your eating.

Next, focus on protein—mainly on the protein in beans and other legumes, fish and soy products.

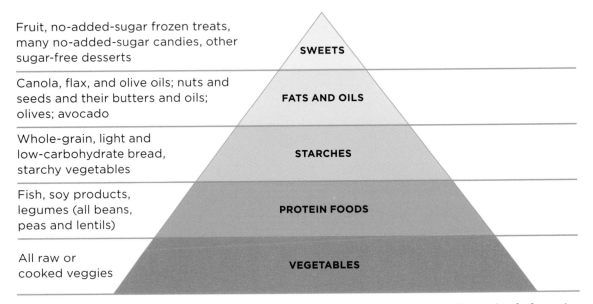

Fruit, no-added-sugar frozen treats, many no-added-sugar candies, other sugar-free desserts — **SWEETS**

Canola, flax, and olive oils; nuts and seeds and their butters and oils; olives; avocado — **FATS AND OILS**

Whole-grain, light and low-carbohydrate bread, starchy vegetables — **STARCHES**

Fish, soy products, legumes (all beans, peas and lentils) — **PROTEIN FOODS**

All raw or cooked veggies — **VEGETABLES**

The next level up is starches—preferably starchy vegetables or breads that are whole grain, light or low carbohydrate. Think of the starches as accompaniments or side dishes rather than the main focus of the meal.

Where fats and oils are concerned, choose canola, flax and olive oils, and eat nuts, seeds, olives and avocado.

For sweet treats, go for fruit and certain products with no added sugar.

We'll tell you much more about the extensive and varied range of options for each level of the Beat Diabetes Pyramid in its own chapter. Suffice it to say that there's nothing particularly complicated about "eating the Pyramid way," as we like to call it. It's pretty simple and straightforward, although, as you'll see in the chapters that follow, it presents an almost dizzying array of food choices and a spectacular range of recipes.

Certainly, the mainstay of eating the Pyramid way is the focus on vegetables and healthy proteins. But no food is forbidden, and we never tell you what to eat or what not to eat. It's a matter of choice, and the choice is yours. What we might suggest, however, if you're a meat lover, a cheese freak or someone who can't resist scrambled eggs for Sunday brunch, is simply that you adjust your thinking a bit and relegate some of those favorites to the category of foods you eat less frequently or less of. Let's say you're a meat-and-potatoes kind of guy. No problem: just maybe try to make meat the side dish and perhaps accompanied by lentils and even a salad with a delicious olive-oil-and-vinegar dressing. It's a matter of emphasis: in featuring the potatoes accompanied by lentils, salad and other vegetables, you're putting your emphasis on the kind of healthy weight loss that will help you beat diabetes.

THE FOUR PHENOMS: YOUR SECRET WEAPON

But there's a secret weapon inside the Beat Diabetes Pyramid as well. Four secret weapons, in fact. We call them the Four Phenoms. The reason? They represent four groups of nutrients that play a pretty prodigious role not just in controlling diabetes but in beating it—in literally helping to reverse its effects. The four are:

- Fiber
- Phytonutrients
- Soy protein
- Good fats

Here's a look at what each is and what it does for your health:

Fiber

Fiber is the structural component of plants. It's a very, very complex carbohydrate that cannot be digested. In Europe, in fact, it isn't counted as a carbohydrate—something to keep in mind if you're reading nutrition labels on your next trip to Paris or Rome.

All edible plants—vegetables, beans, grains and fruits—contain fiber. There is no fiber at all in meat, poultry, seafood, dairy foods, eggs or fats.

There are two main types of fiber: soluble and insoluble. As the names suggest, soluble fiber partially dissolves in water; insoluble fiber does not. Both types of fiber are a real boon for people trying to lose weight because fiber foods make you feel full. The reason is simply that fiber has bulk and takes up space in the intestines; you feel sated, tend to eat less and therefore take in fewer calories. In addition, a lot of high-fiber foods are themselves low in calories, require more chewing and are simply digested more slowly. All of those factors help to diminish your calorie intake, which is the basic requirement for weight loss.

But fiber does even more. Precisely because it slows digestion, fiber retards the process by which sugar enters the bloodstream, thus reducing blood glucose spikes and helping to maintain insulin levels. It also lowers blood pressure, total cholesterol, LDL cholesterol and triglycerides, thus in turn reducing the risk of heart disease—a central consideration given that 80 percent of deaths among diabetics are from cardiovascular failure.

All fiber food sources provide all these benefits, so it is little wonder that fiber figures so prominently in the Beat Diabetes Pyramid. But, as you'll learn in more detail in Chapter 6, some high-fiber foods are also high in calories and therefore will have to be taken in moderation.

Fiber is the one diabetes-beating phenom for which there is a recommended daily amount. Experts say that to get the optimal benefit of fiber's weight loss and disease-fighting power, aim for at least 25 to 30 grams of fiber a day. What constitutes 25 to 30 grams of fiber? This chart will help give you an idea.

FIBER FOOD	AMOUNT	FIBER GRAMS
Lentils, cooked	1 cup	16
Split peas, cooked	1 cup	16
Roasted soy nuts	½ cup	16
Veggie burger, grilled	5 ounces	10
Figs, dried	4	10
Mixed berries, raw	1 cup	8
Apple (skin on), raw	1 medium	5
Carrots, raw	1 cup	5
Spinach, cooked	1 cup	5
Shredded wheat	2 biscuits	5
Sweet potato, baked	1 medium	4
Avocado	½ cup	4
Brown rice, cooked	1 cup	4

But the truth is, if you eat the Beat Diabetes Pyramid way—that is, if you follow the guidelines it represents—you are likely to get all the fiber you need to achieve and maintain a healthy weight.

FIBER AND WEIGHT LOSS

A meta-analysis of studies on increasing fiber found that an additional 14 grams per day resulted in a 10 percent decrease in calorie intake and a weight loss of nearly five pounds over a four-month period.

Phytonutrients

Phytonutrients, as their name suggests, are nutrients found in plants. Actually, to be precise, they are not really nutrients; that is, they're not substances essential for life, like proteins, vitamins, minerals, carbohydrates and water. Instead, what phytonutrients do is toughen the cells of the plants, interacting in complex ways to counter stress, toxins and deterioration. They do the same inside humans, which is why they promote health and advance healing—primarily by defending the cells of the body from damage.

So far, scientists have identified some two thousand phytonutrients. You've probably heard the names of many of them—like the *lycopene* in tomatoes and the *beta-carotene* in carrots. But chances are you've never heard of—and may find difficult to pronounce—*zeaxanthin*, a carotenoid found in leafy greens that helps protect vision, or *daidzein*, an isoflavone found in soy products and a powerful cancer fighter. Yet these tongue-twisting substances—often responsible for the vivid colors of the fruits and vegetables from which they derive—are a key reason why a diet that emphasizes plant-based foods is such a powerful tool for fighting infection and for strengthening your vitality and well-being.

Where diabetes is concerned, the power of phytonutrients is particularly important, for it is well known that many of the complications of diabetes result from damage to the body's blood vessels, large and small, and phytonutrients are powerhouses of blood vessel protection. For example, the phytonutrients in red wine, called *polyphenols*, may relax the artery walls and raise HDL cholesterol. The *allicin* found in onions and garlic can both raise HDL cholesterol and lower LDL cholesterol.

The *genistein* and *phytosterols* that come from soy reduce the formation of plaque in the arteries, and the *coumarins* found in cucumbers, squash, melons, parsley and citrus fruit prevent platelets from sticking together to form a clot or thrombosis, which is often the immediate cause of a heart attack.

Phytonutrients also fight inflammation, which, in the arteries, increases the risk of cardiovascular disease and stroke. In fact, the intake of phytonutrients is inversely related to the formation of C-reactive protein—as mentioned, a key measure of inflammation—so the more phytonutrients you ingest, the less C-reactive protein you are likely to form.

A FLAVONOID FAVOR

If you like the taste of either apples of onions—or both—you're doing yourself a favor. Researchers have found that people who eat foods high in quercetin, a flavonoid antioxidant found in both foods, had a 21 percent lower risk of mortality from cardiovascular disease and were 19 percent less likely to have type 2 diabetes. You can also find quercetin in grapes, tea and citrus fruits.

KEEPING YOUR ARTERIES FLEXIBLE

The power of soybean phytonutrients to help blood flow through the arteries has been well demonstrated in an Australian research study. The study focused on arterial compliance—the technical term for the capacity of large arteries to stretch and bend in response to changes in pressure and volume. Obviously, flexible arteries do far better than stiff arteries in preventing coronary problems, and the Australian research documented how soybean isoflavones improve arterial compliance—that is, they help keep the arteries flexible and thus help keep heart disease at bay.

Perhaps above all, phytonutrients act as antioxidants. In fact, that's probably why they evolved—as defense mechanisms against the free radicals of unstable oxygen that can threaten plant life. Free radicals, of course, are the loose cannons of the cellular world, unstable molecules that can damage cells by destroying the cell membrane. That's what they do to plants, and they can do the same to humans—where diabetes is an issue, they specifically do it to human blood vessels. Yet the antioxidant properties of phytonutrients can inhibit the oxidation of LDL cholesterol in the blood, and since oxidized LDL cholesterol is much more likely to form artery-blocking plaque, preventing its oxidation is as important as—if not more important than—lowering the amount of LDL cholesterol.

In short, these health-promoting substances in plant foods can greatly decrease the risk of cardiovascular disease and other blood vessel damage so common in diabetics. How can you be assured of getting an ample supply of phytonutrients? That's easy. Follow the guidelines of the Beat Diabetes Pyramid.

SOY MILK AND BLOOD PRESSURE

Soy milk—and specifically the phytonutrient genistein, found in soy—has been significantly linked to lowering blood pressure. A three-month, double-blind study of forty men and women with mild to moderate hypertension found that those taking soy milk lowered their systolic blood pressure by 18.4 mm Hg on average and their diastolic blood pressure by 15.9 mm Hg on average—significant reductions for heart health.

Here are some key phytonutrients that help decrease the risk of cardiovascular disease—and here's where to find them.

PHYTONUTRIENT	FOOD SOURCE
Carotenoids	Cantaloupe, carrots, winter squash, pumpkin, sweet potatoes
Lycopene	Tomatoes, red grapefruit, watermelon
Lutein, zeaxanthin	Spinach, kale, turnip greens
Capsaicin	Red chile peppers
Genistein, daidzein	Soybeans and soy products
Anthocyanins	Red and purple grapes, red cabbage, radishes
Anthoxanthins	Cauliflower, potatoes
Betacyanin	Beets
Flavonoids	Citrus fruit, berries, tomatoes, peppers
Lignans	Flaxseeds

BERRY HEALTHY

Berries are rich in polyphenols, and polyphenols are powerful fighters against the risk of cardiovascular disease, as a recent study documented. Study participants consumed a couple of servings of berries each day for two months. At the end of the two months, researchers found favorable changes in platelet function, a decrease in blood pressure and a 5.2 percent increase in levels of HDL cholesterol among the berry eaters, versus a 0.6 percent rise in HDL in the control group.

Soy Protein

If you want to give your heart health a real boost—and deal a knockout punch to diabetes into the bargain—you can't do better than soy protein, found today in a range of products from veggie burgers to "chicken" nuggets, from edamame served as cocktail munchies to Asian dishes focused on bean curd, from smoothies to protein bars for athletes.

Of course, the soybean has been cultivated and used for thousands of years in Asia, and soy protein, as the name suggests, is the protein heart of the plant. What's special about soy protein is that it is what nutritionists call a "complete" protein, containing all the amino acids that we need to obtain through the food we eat because they can't be synthesized in the body. Animal products also offer complete protein, but they contain the kind of fat, especially saturated fat, that can harm heart health and make it tough to maintain a healthy weight.

As a diabetes fighter, soy protein has no match. There are four main ways that soy protein can help you beat diabetes:

1. It helps regulate glucose and insulin levels.
2. It proactively advances weight loss.
3. It lowers the risk of cardiovascular disease and its severity.
4. It lowers the risk and slows the progression of kidney disease, a major complication of diabetes and one to which diabetics are particularly prone.

Let's take them one at a time.

Glucose and insulin levels. Although we're not sure why, studies have shown that diets containing moderate amounts of soy protein can slow the absorption of glucose into the bloodstream, reduce insulin levels and improve insulin resistance. What do we mean by "moderate amounts"? Anywhere from 25 to 40 grams a day, equivalent to two to three servings of any of the soy products we talk about in this book.

In one of the most important studies confirming this powerful capability of soy protein, the study authors worked with two groups of volunteers with type 2 diabetes. All the volunteers took similar medications and in similar amounts. The difference was in their diet. The first group was given a diet in which the protein content consisted of one-third animal protein, one-third soy protein and one-third vegetable protein. Group 2 ate 70 percent animal protein and 30 percent vegetable protein. The test lasted for four years.

At the end of the four years, members of Group 1, the group that ate soy protein in addition to animal and vegetable protein, had reduced their fasting plasma glucose—that's glucose measured after a fast—by 20 mg/dL, reduced their LDL cholesterol by 2 mg/dL and knocked

PEPTIDE POWER

Homing in on some of the interactions that produce the metabolic dynamics of soy protein, researchers have isolated a soy peptide (a peptide is a compound left after protein molecules have been split) called Hinute. Volunteers following a Hinute-enriched diet for eight weeks lost between 4 percent and 7 percent of their body weight. Other studies have shown that other soy peptides also have this specific ability to decrease body fat and cholesterol without causing a decrease in body protein, or lean body mass.

SOY FOR THE HEART

A meta-analysis of results from thirty-eight clinical trials involving more than seven hundred subjects found that an average of 47 grams of soy protein per day reduced total cholesterol by nearly 10 percent, decreased LDL cholesterol by nearly 13 percent and lowered triglyceride levels by 11 percent. Translation? A 20 percent reduction in the risk of heart attack.

25 mg/dL off their serum triglyceride levels. Group 2 participants experienced minimal reductions in these heart-harmful substances—and in some cases even registered gains.

Moreover, the group that ate soy protein also lost significantly less protein in the urine—a sign that their kidneys were functioning better than the kidneys of Group 2 participants.

Weight loss. Soy protein helps people lose weight in two ways: through direct impact on the metabolism—by burning body fat and not lean body protein—and by increasing the sense of satiety so you actually eat less and thus, by definition, take in fewer calories. A number of studies have confirmed these facts.

In one, volunteers who substituted soy foods for an equal amount of meat and dairy lost significantly more weight while keeping lean body mass. In another, two groups of volunteers were placed on formula diets, each containing similar amounts of protein, fat and calories. But in one formula the protein was soy-based, while in the other it was milk-based. The soy group lost significantly more body fat—and dropped their cholesterol levels as well. In a study published in the *European Journal of Clinical Nutrition,* half the participants included some 25 grams of soy per day in their diet; the other half ate no soy. After twelve weeks, the group that ate soy had lost three times more than the non-soy group—16 pounds, a healthy weight loss for the three-month period.

At the same time, soy protein has been demonstrated to stimulate the release of a natural intestinal hormone called cholecystokinin (CCK) that slows down digestion and induces satiety. The result? You feel full, and your calorie intake goes down. And so, of course, does your weight.

Cardiovascular disease. Soy protein helps lower blood pressure, cholesterol, C-reactive protein and triglycerides—all factors that can endanger your cardiovascular system.

Two major studies on men and women documented soy protein's effectiveness in lowering blood pressure. Participants who consumed 25 to 40 grams of soy protein per day lowered their systolic blood pressure by five points and their diastolic pressure by two and a half points.

It is thought that these results were due, in part, to soy's antioxidant properties and to its beneficial effects on inflammation, for both oxidative stress and inflammation are key culprits in hypertension and cardiovascular disease.

In another study, a diet that substituted soy protein for animal protein had a more beneficial effect on both total and LDL cholesterol than a standard low-fat diet. Researchers at the University of Toronto found that a diet high in soy protein and low in saturated fat was as effective as statin drugs in reducing levels of LDL cholesterol and C-reactive protein—that key marker for inflammation and a major risk factor for heart trouble.

Yet another study tracked two groups of volunteers who were given formula diets similar in all but protein content. The group eating soy-based protein had significantly lower levels of total and LDL cholesterol than the group eating milk protein.

Kidney disease. It's one of the most serious complications of diabetes, and, unfortunately, it can be all too common. Some 40 percent of patients starting dialysis have diabetes; an even scarier statistic is that approximately 30 percent of diabetics will develop kidney disease— nephropathy, to give it its official name. Yet the research shows that soy protein can help you avoid this very real danger. Here's why.

Protein increases the workload of the kidneys—which is why so many people with impaired kidney function are put on a low-protein diet. What scientists have now learned is that **the type of protein you take in is more important than the amount of protein in affecting kidney function.** Studies show that substituting soy protein for animal protein may actually help prevent and treat diabetic nephropathy.

The reason? It's soy's ability to improve both the health of the kidney's blood vessels and the composition of the blood. It does this in four basic ways: by lowering total and LDL cholesterol and triglycerides and decreasing oxidation of LDL, by decreasing inflammation in

SOY PROTEIN IMPROVES KIDNEY FUNCTION

In one study, three groups of type 2 diabetics with kidney disease were put on three different diets: a low-protein diet, a high-soy diet and a diet high in milk-based protein. Kidney function was measured by urine albumin excretion (UAE). That's an important gauge of kidney function: the higher the UAE, the worse the kidney function. Here's what the results of the study showed: the low-protein group had no significant reduction in UAE, the soy group reduced UAE by an impressive 9.5 percent and the milk-based-protein group increased UAE by 11.1 percent—a very substantive increase in a very harmful measure.

the arteries, by lowering blood pressure and by decreasing platelet aggregation along with the clot formation that can result. The net effect of all this is that soy protein helps unblock the arteries and improve the flow of blood through the kidneys. In fact, studies on type 2 diabetics show repeatedly that even a moderate incorporation of soy protein can decrease the risk of developing kidney disease and slow the progression of already existing kidney dysfunction.

Bottom line: if you're diabetic, prediabetic or eager to avoid diabetes through weight loss, you want to incorporate adequate amounts of soy protein in your diet. The best way to do that? Follow the guidelines of the Beat Diabetes Pyramid.

Good Fats

We call them "good" fats to distinguish them from those that raise cholesterol, triglycerides, C-reactive protein and insulin resistance in general. You know the ones we mean: the saturated fats and trans fats that are always so much in the news—and which you can read about in the sidebar as well.

Good fats, by contrast, are the monounsaturated, polyunsaturated and omega-3 fats that do just the opposite: they lower cholesterol and may decrease insulin resistance—along with other benefits. The monounsaturated fats found in olive oil, peanut oil, canola oil and nuts and the polyunsaturated fats found in corn oil, safflower oil and sunflower oil—also called omega-6 oils—all decrease both total and LDL cholesterol levels. The polyunsaturates do so to a greater extent than the monounsaturates, but they may actually lower HDL cholesterol a tiny bit. The monounsaturates have no effect on HDL cholesterol, and they may decrease insulin resistance. So both types are good fats that fit in any healthful diet.

The omega-3 fats are a branch of polyunsaturated fats. They are powerful tools for lowering triglycerides; they also lower total and LDL cholesterol, raise HDL cholesterol and

---

"BAD" FATS

Saturated fats are the fats found in meat, poultry, dairy, eggs and palm oil. They make it difficult for insulin receptors to work well, thus lowering their effectiveness and raising the risk of diabetes. Trans fats do the same: they also decrease the body's ability to burn fat, may lower HDL cholesterol even as they raise LDL cholesterol and can increase the levels of C-reactive protein. Half of the trans fats in our American diet come from beef, butter and milk. The other half come from the hydrogenated vegetable oils used to make stick margarines, solid shortenings and all sorts of commercially processed pastries, crackers and fried foods.

decrease blood pressure and blood clot formation. The omega-3s may also reduce resistance to the hormone leptin, which helps regulate appetite and metabolism; anything that boosts your leptin level is a plus for weight loss. In addition, omega-3s may turbocharge the body's fat-burning mechanism. What's more, if you're overweight, a diet high in omega-3s and low in saturated fats may reduce the risk that impaired glucose tolerance will morph into full-blown type 2 diabetes. That makes them powerful diabetes fighters indeed. You can find omega-3s in such foods as flaxseeds and flax oil, fatty fish, walnuts, canola oil, soy oil and salba (see sidebar on page 16).

The polyunsaturated omega-6 oils—corn, safflower and sunflower—are, as mentioned, all good at lowering cholesterol. But a high ratio of omega-6s to omega-3s can actually increase inflammation and raise the risk of cardiovascular dysfunction. How can you be sure your ratio isn't too high? Just follow the guidelines laid out in Chapter 7, "Fats and Oils."

Every diet needs fat. To beat diabetes and its complications, make sure your diet is low in saturated fats, trans fats and cholesterol and that it includes ample amounts of monounsaturated and polyunsaturated fats. One way to be sure: eat the Beat Diabetes Pyramid way.

A FISH STORY YOUR BLOOD WILL APPRECIATE

Think of a blood clot as a papier-mâché creation. The shredded newspaper is provided by fibrinogen, long strands of protein that circulate in your bloodstream, while the glue that holds the strands together is your blood platelets. Sometimes, under certain conditions, the fibrinogen can become entangled with the platelets—and with other elements—and the result is a clot, officially known as a thrombus. So the more fibrinogen in your bloodstream, the higher your risk of clotting and of the consequences clotting can bring. In fact, a recent survey showed that people with high levels of fibrinogen had five times the normal risk of heart attack, recurrent heart attack and premature death.

Enter omega-3 fish oils. They keep unwanted clots from forming in two ways. First, they make your platelets less "gluey" and thus less likely to stick together. Second, they decrease the production of fibrinogen. End result? A greatly reduced risk of a heart attack.

GOT THE PICTURE?

It's really pretty simple. The secret to beating diabetes is healthy weight loss, and the secret to healthy weight loss is eating. Specifically, it's eating in a way that will ensure you defend yourself against insulin resistance and everything that causes it—in other words, getting the nutrients you need to battle metabolic syndrome proactively.

Bottom line: a diet that is low in saturated fats and trans fats, that includes ample amounts of soy protein and focuses on the phytonutrients and fiber of plant-based foods—emphasizing

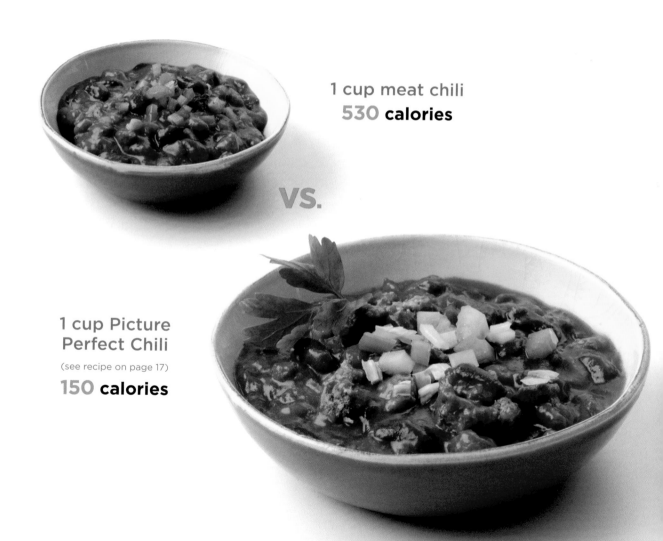

1 cup meat chili
530 calories

VS.

1 cup Picture
Perfect Chili
(see recipe on page 17)
150 calories

AZTEC ENERGY

Among the Aztecs, whose civilization dominated Central America hundreds of years ago, the only way to get word from one village to the next was on foot. That's why Aztecs were such superb runners, and it's why they relied so much on salba, which they referred to as their "running food," believing it gave them energy and power.

They were right. Salba is a grain and a member of the mint family. Its botanical name is *salvia hispanica*, and the ancient Aztecs, like their present-day descendants, cultivated salba and treasured it, even offering it in annual tribute to their rulers.

Today, you can find salba in health stores and organic markets as whole seeds or ground meal. Just one tablespoon contains approximately 2 grams of omega-3 fatty acids—a whole day's worth. And salba is also an excellent source of both fiber and antioxidants. We make no claim as to what it may do to your running skills, but it may just give you the same kind of energy and power it gave the ancient Aztecs.

these ingredients in favor of those that raise cholesterol, increase insulin resistance and retard weight loss—is a diet that can keep you thin and healthy for life.

Take another look at this Picture Perfect Beat Diabetes demonstration. It shows you everything you need to know about this food's power on defense and offense as discussed on pages 1 and 2. As you go through the levels of the Beat Diabetes Pyramid chapter by chapter, and as you study demo after demo, you'll quickly learn the role of different foods in your fight for healthy weight loss. You'll come to understand how the foods you love and the dishes you'd like to try can become your "partners" in arriving at and maintaining the weight you want for the health you deserve. Pretty soon, the knowledge will become automatic—and so will the healthy weight loss.

But first, it's important to remind yourself why you're making these healthy choices.

SMALL CHANGES, BIG IMPACT

Studies have shown that as little as 3 grams per day of two particular omega-3 acids, EPA and DHA, found mostly in fish, can lower your systolic blood pressure by five points and your diastolic pressure by three points. This decrease in blood pressure would reduce the number of Americans with hypertension by 40 percent—a big difference from a little change! Another omega-3 acid, ALA—found in flaxseeds and flax oil, walnuts, canola oil and soy oil—can also lower blood pressure. In fact, a 1 percent increase in blood levels of ALA is linked with a five-point reduction in blood pressure.

PICTURE PERFECT CHILI

1 cup coarsely chopped bell peppers, any color

1 cup chopped onion

3-4 garlic cloves, minced

1 tablespoon olive or canola oil

1 12-ounce package veggie crumbles*

1 15-ounce can black or red beans, drained

1 15-ounce can chili beans in sauce

1 15-ounce jar tomato-based pasta sauce

1 14-ounce can diced tomatoes

1 4- or 5-ounce can chopped green chiles

1 tablespoon chili powder

1 tablespoon oregano

½ teaspoon cumin

1. Sauté peppers, onions and garlic in oil in a large skillet or saucepan over medium-high heat for 2 minutes.

2. Stir in veggie crumbles and cook for another 2 minutes.

3. Add all remaining ingredients and stir well. Bring to a boil, reduce heat to medium-low, cover pan and simmer for 20 minutes, stirring occasionally.

Yield: about ten 1-cup servings;

approximately 150 calories per serving.

*Recipe tested with Morningstar Farms®
Meal Starters™ Grillers Recipe® Crumbles

CHAPTER 2

For Parents: A Warning and a Call to Action

There's a good one-word reason for making the kind of healthy choices embodied in the Beat Diabetes Pyramid: **kids.**

Your kids, if you're a parent. Kids in general, if you're a concerned citizen and taxpayer worried about the rising tide of ill health in this country and the scarily rising cost of health care.

Check out the nearest playground. Those adorable little tykes on the swings and jungle gym are part of the first generation of Americans expected to have a shorter life span than that of their parents. Shorter and sicker.

Look closer. Some of those adorable little tykes are overweight. We used to think of it as charmingly pudgy baby fat. But today we know better. Childhood obesity has become an epidemic in this country, and it is an epidemic with alarming consequences. The extra pounds on little children put them at risk for:

• Heart disease	• Gallstones	• Liver disease	• Joint problems
• Asthma	• Digestive disorders	• Headaches	• Vision problems

That extra weight also increases their risk of diabetes. In fact, *carrying even eleven extra pounds can double an individual's risk of type 2 diabetes.*

What is particularly frightening is that these health problems are showing up earlier and earlier in younger and younger children. *The correlation—obesity and poor health—is now inescapable. Today, almost one in five American four-year-olds is obese. And type 2 diabetes is today being found frequently in children ages eleven and twelve and has been diagnosed in children as young as four.* The link could not be clearer.*

Contracting diabetes before the age of forty shortens life span by some eleven to fourteen years, so when we hear that one-third of everyone born in the year 2005 will get diabetes at some point, it becomes clear why this generation has a shorter life expectancy than the previous

* *Wall Street Journal*, May 19, 2009.

generation. Moreover, in fifteen or twenty years, these kids will be having their own children, to whom they will pass on their unhealthy eating habits. How early will those kids get sick? And what will their life expectancy be?

Excess weight in young children is therefore not cute. With 90 percent of overweight kids having at least one avoidable risk factor for heart disease, an overweight or obese child is a time bomb waiting to go off. Young children who develop type 2 diabetes have more time to accumulate vascular and nerve damage; they are thus more likely to suffer severe and costly complications as they grow to maturity. They will pay a terrible toll in suffering and in limitations to their lives.

And the rest of us will pay a terrible toll in health care costs and in the cost of lost productivity of these individuals.

> ## SODA AND THE METABOLIC SYNDROME
>
> Researchers who tracked some nine thousand men and women over four years concluded that drinking at least one soda per day raised the likelihood of a diagnosis of metabolic syndrome by 44 percent.

THE PSYCHOLOGICAL TOLL

There's another terrible price that children pay for being overweight: it is psychologically painful in a way that can scar an individual for life. Overweight kids often seem "different" or "other" to small children, and they may be made to feel that way: the last kid picked for the team, or the only one not invited to the sleepover. What's more, children—even very young children—can be cruel, and a teasing nickname can slice a child like a knife through the heart.

Ostracized by contemporaries or self-isolated as a defense mechanism, overweight children early on develop a sense of inferiority and feelings of insecurity and low self-esteem, which can affect their adulthood in unhappy ways. In an era when body image seems shaped by impossible magazine fantasies and starved-looking Hollywood starlets on the red carpet, it's little wonder that anorexia, bulimia and other eating disorders are on the rise among children as young as elementary school age, while there is also an increasing and intensifying surge in depression showing up in overweight and obese children. It is a heavy price for a little child to pay during the all-important developmental years.

How did it happen? How did our kids get to be this way—overweight, unhealthy and unhappy about it?

PARENTS ARE RESPONSIBLE

Again, there's a simple one-word answer: us.

Sure, there are lots of outside influences on children—even on very young children—urging them to eat "fun" foods that are bad for them. But the dominant influence on kids, especially very young ones, remains their parents.

Children are not born with poor eating habits or the desire to eat unhealthy foods. They learn the eating habits that form their eating tastes from us, their parents. We're the ones who buy the foods our kids eat. The meals we put on the table, the foods we order in or the restaurants we take our kids to establish patterns our kids learn to mimic. It's how they acquire taste—which is a learned experience. That's how and why we are ultimately the teachers of our children's eating habits, and that makes us responsible for their eating future—and the diseases that come from it.

But lately, many parents seem to have begun to abdicate that responsibility. To be fair, the abdication hasn't been by choice. When both husband and wife are working and the kids are busy with all sorts of after-school activities, it's virtually impossible to plan family meals, much less to sit down together as a family to eat one. Result? Kids—and parents—rely more and more on fast food, which is high in carbohydrates, calories and fats. Americans eat 40 percent of their calories outside the home, and consumer spending on fast food has increased eighteen-fold since 1970. Waistlines have grown with the rise in fast food, and 70 percent of kids ages six to eight think fast food is healthier than homemade food. Sure they do: they have the former almost more frequently than the latter.

And the portions tend to be outsized—having nothing to do with what's sufficient for normal growth, fitness and well-being. A **recommended serving** of meat, fish or poultry is 3 ounces; that is what is recommended for good health and nutrition by the U.S. Department of Agriculture, the Food and Drug Administration and the National Institutes of Health. The **typical portion** of meat, fish or poultry that Americans eat is about 8 ounces—nearly three times what is needed and recommended. Today's typical pasta portion is 480 percent bigger than the government recommendation.

LARGE PACKAGE, SMALL SNACK

Studies show that small packages lead to bigger consumption of high-calorie snacks by the weight-conscious. One look at a large bag of, say, potato chips, and folks conscious of weight and body size may grab one or two, then quit—if they even open the package. But the 100-calorie snack packs are so readily seen as "diet aids" that the weight-conscious chow them down with impunity.

When you ordered a hamburger in 1957, you got a 1-ounce patty on a bun, and the whole thing contained 210 calories. When you order a hamburger today, you're eating 6 ounces of food and taking in 618 calories. A side of fries was once 2.4 ounces, totaling 210 calories; today, you get 6.9 ounces and 610 calories.

School lunches aren't much better; like most assembly-line eateries, they tend to offer lots of fried food, thus doubling down on the carbs, calories and fat content kids get in the fast-food places. And the beverage of choice at school as well as at home or in the restaurant tends to be soda—which is nutrition-free and typically loaded with calories. In 1950, American children drank three cups of milk to one soda; in the twenty-first century, that ratio is precisely reversed, with three sodas to a single cup of milk. Each of those sodas contains 150 calories, and all you need to gain 15 pounds a year is 150 calories—that is, a single soda—per day.

True, we can't be responsible for what our children eat when they are not home. And let's face it, we are up against a formidable opponent in the food industry, which spends tens of billions of dollars on advertising to young children, not to mention the indirect "advertising" on Web sites featuring licensed characters, games and the like. In fact, the average American child sees several thousand food advertisements on television each year. And despite the industry's promises to the contrary, most of the advertising focuses on the least nutritious foods. As we learn from an October 2009 study by Yale University's Rudd Center for Food Policy and Obesity, "the least healthy breakfast cereals are those most frequently and aggressively marketed directly to children as young as age two... The researchers' evaluation of cereal marketing, the first such study of its kind, shows pervasive targeting of children across all media platforms and in stores."* The reason is simple: get kids to like this stuff early, and they'll be customers for life. So today's kids are indeed growing up making unhealthy food choices. Did you know that 25 percent of the vegetables eaten in the United States today are french fries?

In addition, as every parent knows, kids are exercising less. By the age of seventeen, today's child has spent 38 percent more time in front of the TV than in school. According to *Time* magazine, every hour of TV a kid averages per day raises his risk of obesity by some 6 percent. We can't totally blame the kids: if they live in big cities, their parents tell them not to play outside because it's too dangerous. If they live in the suburbs, there may not even be a sidewalk inviting them to walk to school. City or suburb, kids' rooms are equipped with a computer, television, Xbox—you name it. Who wants the fresh air of the outdoors, who needs a

* "Kids Spoon-Fed Marketing and Advertising for Least Healthy Breakfast Cereals,"
  Yale University Office of Public Affairs, October 26, 2009.

leg-stretching run across a field, when you can do it all virtually or watch it from the comfort of your bed? No one, which is why most kids today spend from two to four hours in front of some sort of screen every day—and almost no time outside at all.

With too much fast food that is nutrition-free and a minefield for metabolic syndrome and not enough exercise, no wonder there is an epidemic of childhood obesity and a surge of such killer diseases as diabetes.

So yes, you're up against a formidable obstacle in trying to get your kids to make healthy eating choices—a relentless barrage of images, endless chatter, peer pressure and the ever-present convenience factor.

But you're not without resources. As parents, you are the first habit setters, and you can demonstrate the example both at home and in restaurants. You are also the first authority figures, with immense power to teach your children to make the right choices.

Bottom line? Just as we teach our children how not to behave—not to lie or cheat, not to be rude or unfriendly—so also can we teach them what not to eat. And just as we teach them to be honest, polite, considerate of others and responsible, so also can we give them the foundation of healthy eating that will enable them to grow up strong, fit and as protected against disease as possible.

GIVING YOUR KIDS A HEAD START ON HEALTHY EATING

The Beat Diabetes Pyramid is your family's map to healthy eating. And the sooner you start the better. **With type 2 diabetes showing up in eleven-year-olds, and with obesity plaguing four-year-olds, you cannot afford to wait.**

If you are expecting a child or are the parents of a newborn, you can start providing your child the benefits—and pleasures—of varied, nutritious food as soon as the child is weaned and

---

ENVIRONMENT AFFECTS OBESITY

Who is most likely to be obese? Lower-income minorities and people in rural areas of the country. The Centers for Disease Control and Prevention track obesity by race, income and geography and find that African American and Hispanic children are more likely to be overweight than white American kids. More than twice as many kids living below the poverty line are overweight or obese than kids with family incomes above the line. And 16.5 percent of rural kids versus 14.4 percent of urban kids are obese.

Conclusion? Environment defines the choices available—including the eating choices. And adults create the environment for kids.

you have begun to introduce solid foods. If your child is beginning to show evidence of excess weight, you need to intervene now to retrain his or her way of eating.

Whenever you begin, be sure to think of the changes you are making as being about health. If you talk to your child about the change, frame the discussion in just those terms—that the changes are about getting healthy. **Talk about foods not as good or bad but as healthy or unhealthy. Don't prohibit or restrict any foods;** it will backfire. Instead of eliminating the food from your child's eating pattern, you will imbue that food with special importance.

Perhaps the most important first step is for you yourself to **model the eating behavior you want your child to assume.** There is no more powerful lesson for your child than seeing you enjoy healthful foods and physical activity.

In fact, it is a good idea to **make any change in eating habits a family affair.** Involve everyone in creating a weekly healthy eating plan, and make meals regular collective events— no different meals or special foods for different family members. *Make the outing to a fast-food restaurant a less and less frequent event—*maybe cut back to once a week, then once a month and so on.

MODEL BEHAVIOR

As the song says, children are watching—and researchers at Dartmouth College agree. They took 120 kids ages two to six on a simulated shopping trip. When asked to "buy" foods at the make-believe grocery store stocked with toy foods, children whose parents customarily made healthier food purchases bought healthier foods.

Interview with Jonathan, 13 years old

When Jonathan came to me, he was 12 years old, 5'6" and weighed 228 pounds. Now Jonathan is 13, and after following a new diet for just 21 weeks he has brought his weight down to 186 pounds and significantly improved his health.

Dr. S: What is the main trigger that got you to start a diet?

Jonathan: I would get tired fast. I wanted to do all the things the boys in my class could do. I couldn't exercise the same way as all of them. Now that I've lost weight I am starting on the basketball team. Probably the track team, too. And I'll be able to run more.

Dr. S: What was the most difficult thing about starting a diet?

Jonathan: Not giving up. I didn't give up. I used to eat a lot of fast food and starch, high-calorie foods. I don't eat those foods that often anymore.

Dr. S: Do you miss them?

Jonathan: Sometimes. I have some replacements.

Dr. S: What are the replacements?

Jonathan: I used to have regular sausages—now I have Morningstar sausages. I found healthier snacks—like soy chips and low-calorie popsicles.

Dr. S: Did you ever feel uncomfortable about the fact that you were dieting while the other kids were eating high-calorie foods?

Jonathan: The other kids were eating pizza and other things in school, but it didn't bother me that much because I knew one of these days I would have more energy and I'd be able to keep up with them.

Dr. S: Was it worth it?

Jonathan: Yes, I have more energy now and I can keep up with my friends.

Dr. S: What was the most difficult part of the diet?

Jonathan: Sticking to it in the "middle," when I was partway through.

Dr. S: What advice might you give to a child who needs to go on a diet?

Jonathan: It might be difficult but it's all worth it in the end.

(Jonathan's mother—Stephanie)

Dr. S: When Jonathan decided to start a diet, was it a conversation you had with him or did he come home and say something?

Stephanie: Jonathan asked me for help. He began to develop a complex, and when he asked me for help that's when I began to do the research for a diet. At his school they had an obstacle course for exercising. He couldn't do it. And he was embarrassed—when he did track he was the slowest. There were a couple of other kids on the team who tried to motivate him, but he knew he wasn't part of it. He was discouraged. So when he came to me and asked me for help, it broke my heart.

Dr. S: How do you feel about it now?

Stephanie: I'm so proud of him. A lot of his friends encouraged him and told him he looked great. There were many times he could have gone off of the diet, but he didn't. His attitude is better—now he wants to try on clothes. I'm really proud of him.

Dr. S: Was it difficult for you to make changes in your home?

Stephanie: I pretty much took control of his diet and everyone in the family supported him. Jonathan's diet consisted mostly of fast-food restaurants—Wendy's, McDonald's—and he ate pretty much everything he wanted to eat. In the beginning it was very hard for me because I had to learn for myself, as well, to buy the proper foods. Shopping was so much different than in the past.

Dr. S: Do you feel responsible for the way he was eating before, when he was gaining the weight?

Stephanie: I feel responsible because he ate what was given to him. A lot of junk food, a lot of high-fat foods, foods that I was brought up on. I fed him what I was accustomed to. So this was a change for both of us. My family as well. We drink Crystal Light now and eat Morningstar sausages and other veggie products. There's food in our house that we never had before. He taught himself as well as the family.

Dr. S: So Jonathan's healthier and responsible for helping everyone in your house to eat healthy and lose weight?

Stephanie: I guess you can say that.

Dr. S: I think I will. What advice would you give to a child who's overweight?

Stephanie: Basically, to seek help and to be a leader. I would tell a mother to go out and seek help not just for her child but for everyone in the family.

Dr. S: At what point would you tell a mother to intervene?

Stephanie: Right away—I'm giving advice already.

When you think about it, what you're really trying to do is introduce new foods and/or flip the ratio of foods in a typical meal. That is, where you once served a large platter of meat and made vegetables a side dish, you now want to focus on the vegetables and relegate the meat to a marginal role in the meal. In introducing new foods, be aware that it may take a kid a dozen, fifteen, even eighteen tries before he or she is willing to embrace a new food. Our advice? Keep bringing the food back over and over again in different guises or versions and just put it on the table.

Suppose you offered green beans one day and they didn't get a great reception. Bring them back the next day in a soup, the next day in a stew, the next day on a pizza, the next day cold in a salad. Keep at it, and don't be discouraged. In time, your child will begin to taste the new food, then to accept it, then to like it.

SNACK ATTACK

Commercials do sell products, which is bad news when so many TV ads are for unhealthy foods. When kids between the ages of seven and eleven were shown a half-hour cartoon interspersed with ads for food, they ate 45 percent more than did kids of the same age who watched the same cartoon with non-food-related ads. Ditto for adults: they snacked more while watching TV shows with ads for junk food than those with ads promoting healthful foods or good nutrition.

Another trick: disguise the healthy food in or as something already well known. Our nutritionist has created recipes for pizza (page 38), a smoothie (page 40) and cookies (page 52) that are actually soy-based—and no one ever realizes it. Dr. Shapiro once served soy sausages to a bunch of New York City firemen, and they scarfed them down with gusto. Serve kids fruit on top of French toast or as a fruit pizza topping, or hide vegetables in a tart, and they'll think these foods are fun to eat.

You'll find plenty of recipes and food comparison demonstrations in these pages that will help you provide healthy foods to your children in varied versions or in clever disguises.

In addition, here are some essential dos and don'ts for building a strong foundation of healthy eating for your children.

Don't:
- Make food a bargaining chip
- Judge your child's eating either in words or body language
- Deprecate your own body image, weight or eating habits in front of your kids
- Pressure your kids—about their appearance, achievements, etc.—such that they flee from the pressure into food
- Isolate your overweight child from his or her siblings
- Force your child to eat when he or she claims satiety or lack of hunger

Do:
- Start early
- Make mealtime as much fun as possible
- Stock your larder with healthy snacks—after cleansing it of high-calorie foods
- Set limits on computer and television time for your kids; two to four hours a day is way too much for bodies that are developing and growing
- Serve small portions; if your child asks for a second helping, offer the lower-calorie foods first

Encourage exercise by taking a walk with your kids, playing catch with them, enrolling them in sports activities. Assign household chores that require movement: mowing the lawn, walking the dog, cycling to the store to pick up a loaf of bread.

Listen to your kids. If your child tells you about an incident of teasing or the like at school or makes negative comments about his or her body, seize the moment to have a discussion about healthy eating as a means to weight loss and strength.

Make sure you lavish the same love and attention on your overweight child as on all your children; they very much need to know they're important to you.

Seek professional help and a thorough medical evaluation for your child if his or her excess weight has you concerned.

DOING IT RIGHT

And when you implement the changes that can save your child from a life of overweight and ill health, be sure to do it right. That means following the Beat Diabetes Pyramid as closely as possible, every day, at every meal.

As you go through the Pyramid chapter by chapter, you'll see precisely why. You'll learn about "light" foods that are anything but, about foods that claim to be "reduced fat" but still offer the wrong kind of fat, about "saboteur" foods that look and sound good for you—natural! wholesome!—but are actually loaded with calories and with substances that raise your risk of metabolic syndrome and your susceptibility to such killer diseases as diabetes.

The following meal plans show you what we mean. The daily meal plan on the left looks and sounds benign enough, but check out the totals compared to the far better meal plan—based on the Beat Diabetes Pyramid—on the right.

It isn't even just a matter of the numbers; it's also a question of the kinds of ingredients. Fats from milk, cheese, turkey, sour cream and sugar-free cookies are the "bad" kind of fat we discussed in Chapter 2. The low-fat granola is full of calories and added sugar. The 2 percent milk isn't much lower in saturated fat than whole milk—not to mention the fact that dairy is not recommended for preventing or managing diabetes. Even the seven-grain bread, which sounds so nutritious, doesn't necessarily contain the whole grain that is so important for nutrition. As to the sugar-free cookies, they are full of starch and fat.

BENIGN?		BETTER	
Breakfast			
1 cup low-fat granola	360 calories, 5 grams fat, 4 grams fiber	1 cup Cheerios	110 calories, 2 grams fat, 3 grams fiber
1 cup 2% milk	130 calories, 5 grams fat, 0 grams fiber	1 cup vanilla soy milk	90 calories, 5 grams fat, 0 grams fiber
		½ cup blueberries	35 calories, 0 grams fat, 4 grams fiber
Total	**490 calories, 10 grams fat, 4 grams fiber**	**Total**	**235 calories, 7 grams fat, 7 grams fiber**

BENIGN?		BETTER	
Lunch			
3 ounces reduced-fat American cheese	220 calories, 13 grams fat, 0 grams fiber	2 tablespoons peanut butter	190 calories, 16 grams fat, 2 grams fiber
2 slices seven-grain bread	180 calories, 2 grams fat, 2 grams fiber	2 tablespoons sugar-free jam	20 calories, 0 grams fat, 0 grams fiber
6 small sugar-free cookies	260 calories, 12 grams fat, 0 grams fiber	2 slices light whole-wheat bread	80 calories, 0 grams fat, 5 grams fiber
		6 dried apricot halves	50 calories, 0 grams fat, 2 grams fiber
Total	**660 calories, 27 grams fat, 2 grams fiber**	**Total**	**340 calories, 16 grams fat, 9 grams fiber**
Snack			
Skinny Cow low-fat ice-cream bar	100 calories, 2 grams fat, 2 grams fiber	Fudgsicle, no sugar added	40 calories, 0 grams fat, 0 grams fiber
Dinner			
1 cup turkey chili	320 calories, 18 grams fat, 1 gram fiber	1 cup three-bean chili	140 calories, 3 grams fat, 9 grams fiber
¼ cup light sour cream	80 calories, 4 grams fat, 0 grams fiber	¼ cup salsa	20 calories, 0 grams fat, 1 gram fiber
Lettuce and tomato	10 calories, 0 grams fat, 1 gram fiber	2 tablespoons guacamole	55 calories, 5 grams fat, 1 gram fiber
Total	**410 calories, 22 grams fat, 2 grams fiber**	**Total**	**215 calories, 8 grams fat, 11 grams fiber**
Daily Total	**1,660 calories, 61 grams fat, 10 grams fiber**	**Daily Total**	**830 calories, 31 grams fat, 27 grams fiber**

Now look how the Beat Diabetes Pyramid would do it, giving your child half the calories, half the fat and more than three times the fiber. This meal plan offers healthy fats from soy milk, peanut butter and guacamole. The classic Cheerios breakfast, as opposed to the granola on the left, includes a whole-grain cereal without added sugar. It's served with soy milk that is low in saturated fat, cholesterol-free and, as you will read in the pages that follow, filled with benefits for weight loss, heart health and diabetes prevention. The sandwich bread is light bread, versus the seven-grain bread used on the left; it is lower in calories than regular bread and is an excellent source of fiber—the same amount of fiber (or more) than you find in regular whole-grain bread.

Get the picture? Then it's time to start doing for yourself and your children what your mother told you time and time again—that is, to eat your vegetables.

FOOD FOR THOUGHT: IT'S YOUR CHOICE

Eating is a matter of choosing. Below are different food options with equal calories. Seeing the difference between food options can help you make healthy choices for a healthier you, and your children.

	Calories	
1 part-skim mozzarella stick	= 85 =	1 cup black bean soup
1 sip lemonade	= 5 =	1 cup diet lemonade
1 Weight Watchers Giant Fudge Bar	= 75 =	4 fruit popsicles, no added sugar
1 serving fries	= 400 =	4 ears of corn
1 wedge apple pie	= 420 =	4 baked apples
1 cup granola	= 550 =	5 cups Cheerios
1 blueberry muffin (6 ounces)	= 540 =	6 light waffles with blueberries and sugar-free syrup
1 individual raspberry tart	= 400 =	8 cups raspberries
1 buttered bagel	= 650 =	14 slices light bread with sugar-free jam
1 cup yogurt pretzels	= 620 =	16 cups popcorn
1 cup superpremium ice cream	= 760 =	19 frozen fudge pops, no added sugar
1 cup orange juice	= 110 =	3 oranges

Want to show your kids how healthy eating can be fun, tasty and important? Sit down with them and go through the food demonstrations that follow. Every kid will find foods to love in these pages, so the demos are a great way to introduce your kids to new food choices—and to the idea that healthy eating is the most satisfying eating there is...

TOTING UP TACO BELL

Stopping by Taco Bell with the kids? Try steering them to the lower-calorie, better-for-you choices—a veggie fajita wrap or bean burrito, both of which offer the benefits of fiber—instead of the supersized nachos, loaded with saturated fat.

Nachos Bell Grande
740 calories

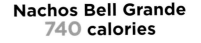

VS.

Veggie Fajita Wrap
420 calories

Bean Burrito
380 calories

CARROT CAKE COUNTDOWN

Just because it has carrots doesn't necessarily mean it's good for you. Take a look at what this slice of carrot cake contains in terms of fat, starch and sugar. That's an 820-calorie danger signal for your health—not to mention the impact on your waistline!

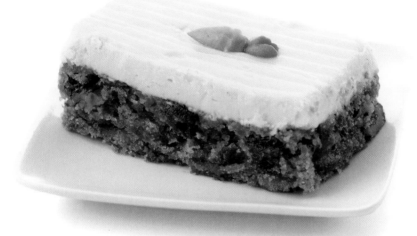

6 ounces carrot cake
820 calories

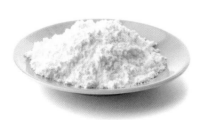
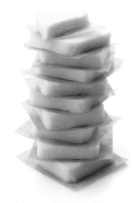
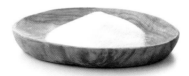

38 grams starch
= 9½ teaspoons

48 grams bad fat
= 9½ pats butter

52 grams sugar
= 13 teaspoons

LUNCH OUT

You're out doing errands, the kids are with you and it's lunchtime. To avoid the chaos and mayhem that hungry children can cause, you've got to feed them on the road. You can do so without sacrificing their health.

Drive right past that fast-food franchise that only offers burgers and head for one that offers more—or for the downtown coffee shop that makes sandwiches to go. Just look at the difference. The typical fast-food cheeseburger lunch, overstuffed with calories and saturated fat, is a ready-made package of future ill health. A more varied lunch—turkey sandwich with fruit and nuts—comes in at half that calorie count, while a tuna salad sandwich plus a banana and diet drink offers even less in the way of calories. Neither of these choices contains saturated fat, and both offer the health benefits of whole wheat and fruit.

You hate it when your kids get hungry and cranky, but you love them enough to make sure you satisfy their hunger in a healthy way.

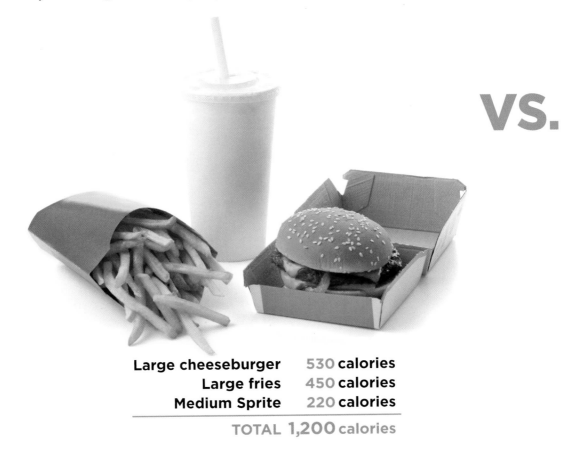

VS.

Large cheeseburger	**530** calories
Large fries	**450** calories
Medium Sprite	**220** calories
TOTAL	**1,200** calories

Tuna salad on whole wheat	395	calories
Banana	100	calories
Diet Sprite	0	calories
TOTAL	495	calories

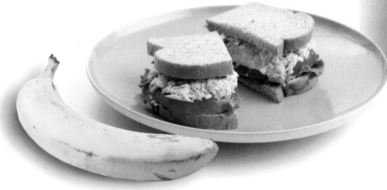

or

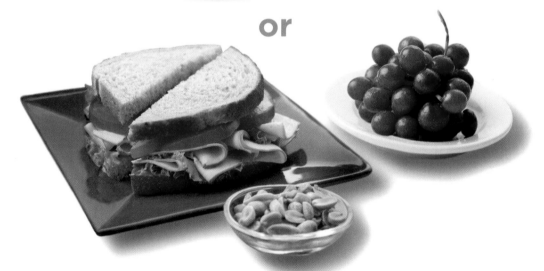

Turkey sandwich on whole wheat with light mayo	440	calories
Grapes	90	calories
Small package peanuts	140	calories
TOTAL	670	calories

MEASURE FOR MEASURE

Here's a difference in weight loss and diabetes-fighting power that's pretty remarkable—especially if you love the taste of salami. Look at the salami sandwich on the left, and note how it measures up in terms of calories and fat. Both measures are pretty stunning. Now check out the sandwich's fiber content: just 2 grams.

Contrast those measures with the measures of the veggie salami sandwich on the right plus a cup of tomato vegetable soup with its healthful supply of phytonutrients. At less than half the calories and only 4 percent of the fat, this lunch is already a help to your waistline and your fight against diabetes. Add in the 10 grams of weight-busting fiber and the soy protein of the veggie salami, and you have a diabetes fighter that really measures up.

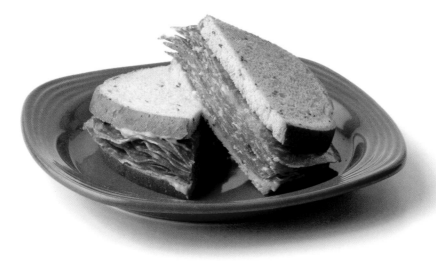

VS.

2 slices rye bread	160 **calories**	0 **grams fat**	2 **grams fiber**
6 ounces salami	540 **calories**	50 **grams fat**	0 **grams fiber**
1 tablespoon mustard	10 **calories**	0 **grams fat**	0 **grams fiber**
TOTAL	710 calories	50 grams fat	2 grams fiber

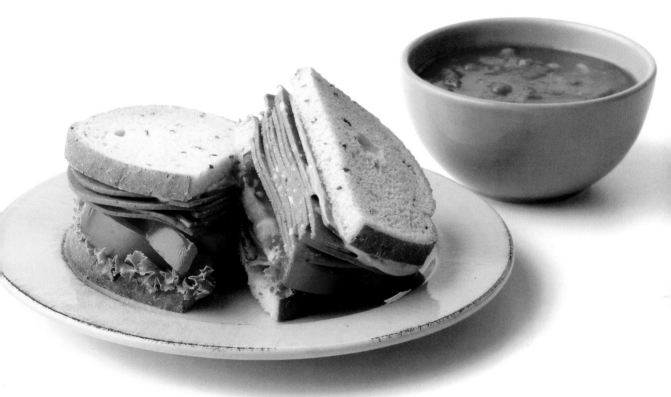

2 slices light rye bread	80 calories	0 grams fat	4 grams fiber
4 ounces veggie salami	140 calories	1 gram fat	2 grams fiber
Lettuce/tomato	10 calories	0 grams fat	2 grams fiber
1 tablespoon mustard	10 calories	0 grams fat	0 grams fiber
1 cup tomato vegetable soup	70 calories	1 gram fat	2 grams fiber
TOTAL	310 calories	2 grams fat	10 grams fiber

A TREAT EVEN A MOTHER CAN LOVE

Sometimes kids just need a treat. (In fact, sometimes everyone needs a treat.) But you can help steer your kids to the kind of treat that has minimal adverse impact on their health. Instead of this chocolate chip cookie, for example, offer your child this frozen yogurt in a cone. Yes, it has some sugar and starch, but at about one-fifth the calories of the cookie and with no fat, it's a treat for parent as well as child.

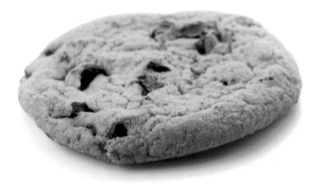

**4-ounce chocolate
chip cookie**
640 calories, 40 grams fat

VS.

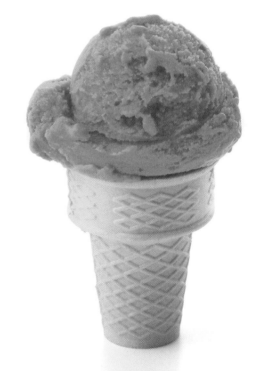

**1 scoop frozen yogurt
with cone**
140 calories, 0 grams fat

PB&J

It's everybody's favorite, but if you're weight-conscious, you can make it with a significant difference in calories that can achieve a significant difference for your waistline *and* your health. Use light bread, which is a great low-calorie source of fiber, and sugar-free jam and save 200 calories. You'll still get all the taste you love—without the high calorie count that doesn't love you.

2 slices wheat bread	**180** calories
2 tablespoons peanut butter	**190** calories
2 tablespoons jam	**120** calories
TOTAL	**490** calories

VS.

2 slices light wheat bread	**80** calories
2 tablespoons peanut butter	**190** calories
2 tablespoons sugar-free jam	**20** calories
TOTAL	**290** calories

37

POLKA DOT PIZZA

1 large low-carb, high-fiber tortilla*

½ cup tomato-based pasta sauce or pizza sauce

½ cup zucchini slices; steamed

2 plum tomatoes, sliced

1 ounce veggie pepperoni slices (12-14 slices)

1 tablespoon chopped herbs—basil, oregano, Italian blend, etc.

Garlic powder

Salt

Pepper

Olive oil

1. **Preheat oven to 500°F. Oil a baking sheet or spray with nonstick spray.**

2. **Place tortilla on baking sheet and spread sauce evenly over top, leaving a ½-inch border.**

3. **Arrange zucchini, tomato and pepperoni slices over sauce.**

4. **Sprinkle herbs on top. Sprinkle on garlic powder, salt and pepper to taste.**

5. **Drizzle with olive oil.**

6. **Bake 10 minutes, or until edges are crisp.**

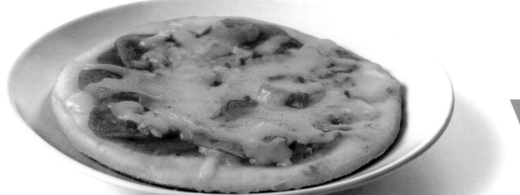

VS.

Pepperoni Pizza
Celeste Pizza-for-One
546 calories, 3 grams of fiber
30 grams of fat = 6 pats butter

*For example, La Tortilla Factory, Whole Wheat Low Carb, or Tumaro's Gourmet Tortillas, Multi-Grain Low Carb.

Polka Dot Pizza
Makes 1 serving
230 calories
20 grams of fiber
7 grams of fat
= 1½ **teaspoons oil**

MAUVE MADNESS

¾ cup blueberries and/or blackberries

¾ cup soy milk

1 teaspoon vanilla or almond extract

3–4 packets Splenda

½ cup crushed ice or a few ice cubes

1. **Process all ingredients except ice in a blender until smooth.**

2. **Add ice gradually, blending well after each addition.**

VS.

8 ounce berry-flavored yogurt
240 calories, 0 grams of fiber
40 grams sugar
= 10 teaspoons sugar

Mauve Madness
Yield: 1 serving
120 calories
6 grams of fiber
0 grams added sugar

PUMPKIN PIE PUDDING

1 15-ounce can pumpkin

1 package sugar-free instant vanilla pudding

¾ cup water

1 tablespoon brandy or rum (optional)

1 teaspoon cinnamon

½ teaspoon pumpkin pie spice

¼ teaspoon salt

Mint leaves

Whipped topping for garnish if desired

1. **Combine all ingredients except mint leaves and whipped topping in a mixing bowl and beat with an electric mixer for about 1 minute, or until smooth and well blended.**

2. **Spoon into dessert dishes and refrigerate at least 30 minutes before serving.**

3. **Garnish with mint leaves and whipped topping, if desired.**

Yield: 4 servings

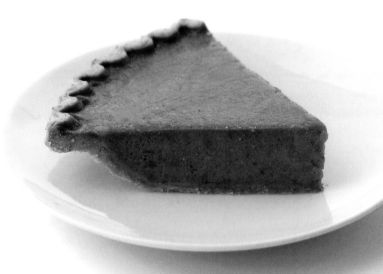

**1 slice pumpkin pie
390 calories, 17 grams of fat,
33 grams of sugar
= 5½ pats butter,
8 teaspoons sugar**

VS.

Pumpkin Pie Pudding
65 calories,
5 grams fiber
0 grams fat,
0 grams sugar

VEGETABLE TART WITH POTATO CRUST

CRUST

1 pound frozen hash brown potatoes, thawed

3 scallions, chopped

¼ cup liquid egg substitute

1 teaspoon finely chopped fresh thyme

¼ teaspoon salt

FILLING

1 small zucchini, chopped

1 garlic clove, minced

2 slices veggie Canadian bacon or 2 veggie bacon strips, chopped

2 cups packed coarsely chopped spinach leaves

1 small tomato, cored and chopped

¼ teaspoon salt

¼ teaspoon freshly ground black pepper

¾ cup liquid egg substitute

¼ cup (1 ounce) shredded fat-free cheddar cheese or dairy-free alternative

Preheat the oven to 350°F. Coat a 9-inch pie plate or tart pan with removable bottom with cooking spray.

1. In a medium bowl, combine the potatoes, scallions, egg substitute, thyme and salt. Press the mixture onto the bottom and up the side of the prepared pan. Bake for 30 minutes, or until firm to the touch. Cool on a rack.

2. Meanwhile, heat a medium nonstick skillet coated with cooking spray over medium heat. Add the zucchini and garlic and cook, stirring, for 2 minutes, or until tender. Add the Canadian bacon, spinach, tomato, salt and pepper and cook, stirring frequently, for 5 minutes, or until the spinach is wilted and the liquid has evaporated. Remove from the heat and cool. Stir in the egg substitute.

3. Pour the vegetable mixture into the crust. Sprinkle with the cheese. Bake for 25 minutes, or until the filling is set and the crust is golden brown.

Yield: 6 servings

Per serving: 140 calories, 2 grams fat

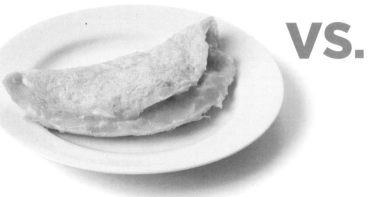

VS.

1 cheese omelet
490 calories, 38 grams fat

Tart for a Start

It would take more than three servings of tart to equal the calorie count of this single cheese omelet. But calories are only part of the story. The omelet, made with two eggs and cheddar cheese and fried in butter, has five times more fat than the tart. What's more, the omelet contains the "bad" saturated fats that raise levels of LDL cholesterol and may increase the risk of heart disease. Start your day instead with nutrient-rich, fiber-filled vegetables in a tasty tart.

3½ servings
Vegetable Tart with Potato Crust
490 calories,
7 grams fat

BEAN BURGERS WITH LIME-SCALLION YOGURT SAUCE

½ cup low-fat plain yogurt or soy alternative

1 scallion, white and green parts, finely chopped

1 teaspoon lime juice

1 15 ½-ounce can black beans, rinsed and drained

1 large egg white or ¼ cup liquid egg substitute

¼ cup chopped fresh cilantro

½ red onion, coarsely grated

1 jalapeño, seeded and finely chopped (wear plastic gloves when handling)

1 tablespoon unseasoned whole-wheat bread crumbs

½ teaspoon cumin

¼ teaspoon garlic salt

4 whole-wheat pitas or lavash breads, warmed

4 large leaves romaine lettuce, shredded

4 thick slices tomato

1. **In a small bowl, combine the yogurt, scallion and lime juice. Chill the sauce until ready to serve.**

2. **In a large bowl, mash the beans with the egg white or egg substitute until only slightly lumpy. Stir in the cilantro, onion, jalapeño, bread crumbs, cumin and garlic salt until well combined. With floured hands, shape the bean mixture into 4 burgers.**

3. **Heat a large nonstick skillet coated with cooking spray over medium heat. Add the burgers and cook for 4 minutes per side, or until lightly browned and firm.**

4. **Place the burgers in the pitas or lavash. Top each with the sauce, lettuce and tomato.**

Yield: 4 burgers

Per burger: 305 calories, 3 grams fat

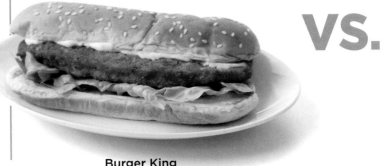

VS.

**Burger King
chicken sandwich
660 calories, 39 grams fat**

Fast-Food Object Lesson

Here's proof, if more were needed, that mass-producing food for speedy delivery and low cost carries a high price tag in calories and saturated fat. And while some fast-food places are opting for low-calorie options, chicken does not necessarily qualify. Instead, go for this quick-to-make bean burger. Flavored with a zesty salsa and wrapped in pita or lavash bread, it's a quick and healthy treat.

Bean Burger
with Lime-Scallion
Yogurt Sauce
305 calories
3 grams fat

FRUIT PIZZA

1 cup light vanilla yogurt or soy alternative

4 light English muffins, split

1 peach

½ cup raspberries

1 teaspoon Splenda

¼ teaspoon cinnamon

1. Line a sieve with 2 pieces of paper towel. Place the sieve over a bowl. Spoon the yogurt into the sieve. Cover with plastic wrap and place in the refrigerator overnight.

2. Preheat the broiler. Cut a peach into segments. Place the English muffin halves on a broiler pan rack. Coat lightly with cooking spray. Sprinkle each muffin half with some of the Splenda and cinnamon. Broil for 1-2 minutes, or until golden brown. Remove the muffin halves. Top with the yogurt and fruit.

Yield: 4 servings (1 whole muffin per serving)

Per serving: **160** calories, **1** gram fat

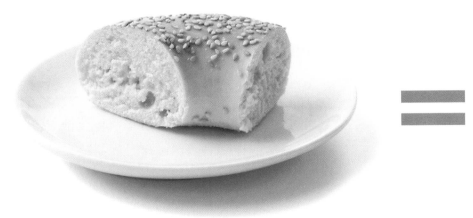

⅓ 6-ounce bagel
160 calories, **1** gram fat

Pizza for Breakfast

Is there a kid who doesn't love pizza? Give yours a change-of-pace treat and concoct this high-nutrition Fruit Pizza for breakfast. It starts with a light English muffin, adds fresh fruit and berries, yogurt as the pizza "cheese," even some cinnamon flavor. A great way to incorporate fruit into your child's diet, a delicious start to the day and a healthful and satisfying alternative to the nutrition-free calories of this piece of bagel.

1 serving Fruit Pizza
160 calories
1 gram fat

STUFFED FRENCH TOAST

1 cup liquid egg substitute

½ teaspoon grated orange peel

8 slices light bread, any flavor

½ cup light cream cheese or nondairy alternative

½ cup sugar-free syrup

½ cup blueberries and/or strawberries

Preheat the oven to 450°F. Coat a baking sheet with cooking spray.

1. In a pie plate, combine the egg substitute and orange peel. Dip each slice of bread into the egg mixture, turning to coat, until each slice has soaked up some batter. Place on the prepared baking sheet. Bake for 12 minutes, turning once, or until golden brown.

2. Spread 2 tablespoons cream cheese on each of 4 slices of the bread. Arrange the strawberries on top. Cover with the remaining bread slices to make 4 sandwiches.

3. To serve, cut each sandwich diagonally in half. Evenly divide the syrup over each sandwich and sprinkle with berries.

Yield: 4 servings

Per serving: 210 calories, 2 grams fat

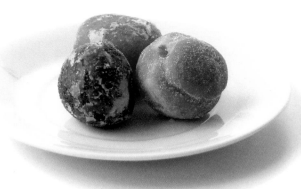

3 doughnut holes
210 calories, 9 grams fat

**1 serving Stuffed
French Toast**
210 calories
2 grams fat

BEAT DIABETES PEANUT BUTTER "COOKIES"

2 scoops unsweetened
soy protein powder (about
²⁄₃ cup)*

²⁄₃ cup granulated Splenda

6 tablespoons creamy
peanut butter

¼ – ⅓ cup chopped peanuts

6 tablespoons water

1 teaspoon vanilla extract

¼ teaspoons salt (if using
unsalted peanut butter, add
an additional pinch of salt)

Preheat oven to 375°F. Lightly oil a baking sheet, or coat
with nonstick spray.

1. In a large bowl, mix all ingredients together until a
dough is formed. If mixture is too dry, add an additional
1 tablespoon water.

2. Roll tablespoons of dough into 1-inch balls and
place on prepared baking sheet; flatten balls into
approximately 2-inch rounds.

3. Bake 8 minutes, or until bottoms are lightly browned.
Cool before removing from pan.

Yield: about 12 cookies

Approx. 78 calories per cookie

BEAT DIABETES ALMOND "COOKIES"

Simply follow the above recipe substituting almond
butter and chopped almonds for the peanut butter and
chopped peanuts, and almond extract for the vanilla
extract.

ATTENTION COOKIE DOUGH LOVERS: this dough is safe
to eat—feel free to sneak a few mouthfuls!

These cookies are a good source of soy protein and
diabetes-friendly monounsaturated fat.

* Available in health-food stores and many markets (Whole Foods, Trader Joe's, etc).

BITE OR BURN

Eating to beat diabetes doesn't mean you can't eat that fast food you've been craving. Exercise also plays an integral role in keeping the disease, and your waistline, at bay. The figures below illustrate just how much exercise it takes to burn off the calories of some of the non-pyramid foods in this chapter.

FOOD	EXERCISE EQUIVALENT
Nachos Bell Grande	1 hour rock climbing or 1.8 hours race walking
Large cheeseburger	5 hours skydiving
Salami sandwich	1 hour jumping rope
Chocolate chip cookie	2 ½ hours dancing or 6.4 trips up and down the stairs of the Statue of Liberty
Peanut butter and jelly sandwich	1 hour cross-country skiing
Celeste Pizza-for-One Pepperoni Pizza	35 minutes swimming + 35 minutes racquetball
Berry-flavored yogurt	32 minutes canoeing or 1 hour 25 minutes ballroom dancing
Pumpkin pie	36 minutes jumping rope
Cheese omelet	1 hour karate
Burger King Chicken Sandwich	32 minutes jumping rope and running up and down the 108 steps of the Philadelphia Art Museum seven times as Sylvester Stallone did in the movie *Rocky*
⅓ bagel	41 minutes raking leaves
3 doughnut holes	21 minutes on StairMaster

CHAPTER 3

The Eat & Beat Diabetes Pyramid

You're about to start climbing the pyramid, one rung at a time, one chapter per rung. For each rung, the chapter will talk about the foods the rung represents and the relative role those foods should play in your overall eating plan if you are to get the most benefit in terms of weight loss and fighting diabetes. Put it all together and eat the way the Pyramid guides you, and you will automatically be doing your utmost to lose weight and fight diabetes.

Let's be clear about one thing: the Pyramid is not a diet. It is not an instruction manual lecturing you on how to put together a meal, how to cook it, how much of it to prepare or when to eat it. Rather, it's the visual embodiment of a healthy way of eating that can keep you slender and free of the effects of diabetes for life.

That means first of all that no food is forbidden. Don't look at the Pyramid and assume that if you follow its guidelines, you have eaten your last serving of hot Italian sausage, your last piece of chocolate cake or your last bag of potato chips. There are moments in life when only potato chips will do, dinners that cry out for chocolate cake at the end, cookouts where the aroma of grilled sausage is just about more than you can bear. Give in. The occasional self-indulgent treat is good for the soul, and what's good for the soul is good for your health.

Second, it means that you don't have to think about including something from every rung of the Pyramid at every meal, or even every day. These rungs don't constitute mathematical proportions to be adhered to with rigorous precision; again, they represent relations among food groups, and the bottom line is indeed that it's all relative, not carved in stone.

Should you count calories? No, although it is absolutely true that calories count. To lose weight, you need to take in fewer calories than you've become accustomed to; to maintain a healthy weight, you need to take in fewer calories than you expend in energy. But if you follow the guidelines of the Beat Diabetes Pyramid, you're already doing that automatically, so you don't need to count calories.

Ditto for portion size. If you're filling up on the Pyramid way of eating—which means plenty of low-calorie foods that contain nutrients and keep you feeling full—portion control is simply not an issue. You'll feel satisfied, even sated, thanks to all the fiber, protein and good taste you'll be enjoying. We promise.

In other words, by following the guidelines represented in the Pyramid, as we explain those guidelines in the chapters that follow, you'll be eating healthier foods, will be decreasing the number of calories you take in and will feel fuller longer without even trying. In other words, you'll be on a really good diet, but it won't feel like one.

Bottom line? Eat when hungry, stop when satisfied. So long as you're eating the Pyramid way, you'll lose weight and fight diabetes successfully with every meal, snack or banquet.

Now, to get you in the mood for climbing the Beat Diabetes Pyramid, we've prepared a quiz to test your Beat Diabetes savvy. You'll find the answers following the quiz. Give yourself one point for every right answer. If you score between 5 and 10, you're pretty savvy, and some of what you read in the next five chapters will be familiar to you. Any score below 5 means you're embarking on a journey of discovery as you turn the pages.

Whatever your score here, you become a real winner when you follow the Pyramid guidelines to weight loss and the prevention and management of this killer disease.

**1. Which is higher in calories—
the mozzarella stick or the ten olives?**

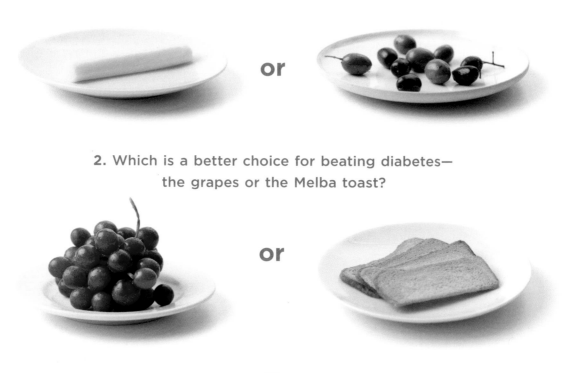

or

**2. Which is a better choice for beating diabetes—
the grapes or the Melba toast?**

or

3. Which is higher in fiber—
the light white bread or the cornflakes?

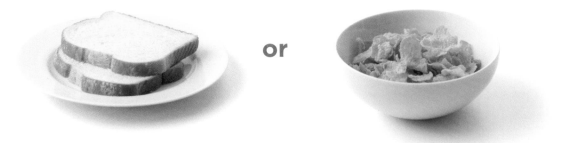

or

4. Which contains more saturated fat—
the avocado or this portion of feta cheese?

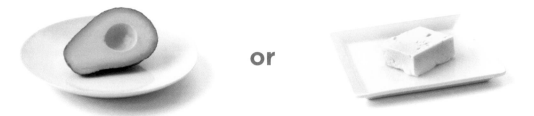

or

5. Which snack has more calories—
this granola bar or the dried apricot halves?

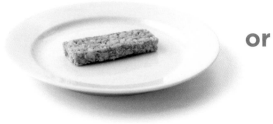

or

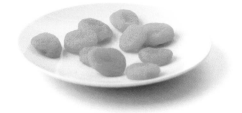

6. Which of these two is more effective in beating diabetes—
the ear of corn or the cup of steamed rice?

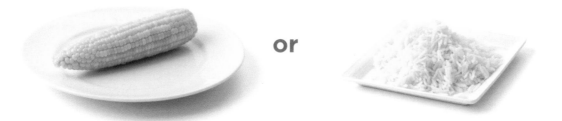

7. Which snack is higher in refined carbohydrates—
pretzel nuggets or jelly beans?

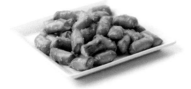 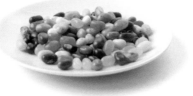

8. Which is higher in saturated fat—
the pistachios or the Muenster cheese?

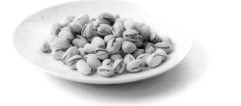 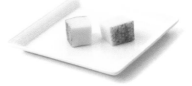

9. Which food should you choose if you're trying to beat diabetes—
the sugar-free cookies or the banana?

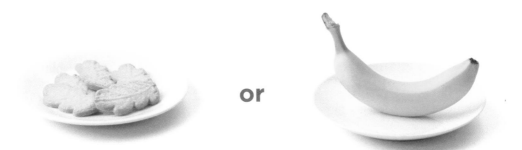

or

10. Which dessert is lower in calories—
Weight Watchers Chocolate Fudge Bar or Tofutti Chocolate Fudge Treats?

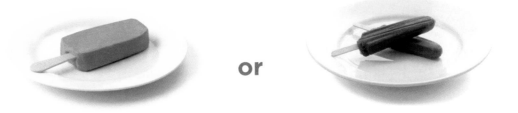

or

ANSWERS:

1. The mozzarella stick, with 90 calories, is almost twice as caloric as the assorted olives, which together have only 50 calories. What's more, the calories in the olives come from "good" or monounsaturated fat—and contain no cholesterol.

2. Both the cup of grapes and the four slices of Melba toast contain 60 calories. But that's just part of the story. The grapes are a good source of phytonutrients and fiber, two of the Four Phenoms, while the Melba toast offers only refined carbohydrates from flour. Go for the grapes.

3. All light breads are good fiber sources, with some 2 to 3 grams of fiber per slice, and that's the situation here: the two slices of light white bread beat the cup of cornflakes for fiber content. The cornflakes, a refined grain product, contain less than a single gram of fiber. Have the bread.

4. With 8½ grams of saturated fat, the feta contains much more than the avocado, which contains only 2 grams of saturated fat. And while the cheese also contains some 50 mg of cholesterol, the avocado has no cholesterol, has "good" fat, 2½ grams of fiber and heart-healthy phytonutrients.

5. The granola bar, small as it is, contains 130 calories and about 20 grams of carbohydrates, mainly from added sugar. The apricots, by contrast, contain a mere 80 calories and are a great source of fiber and phytonutrients.

6. The corn is a better choice. With 4 grams of fiber and 100 calories, it's a healthier bet than the rice, with less than 1 gram of fiber and 200 calories.

7. It's a draw! Both the pretzel nuggets and the jelly beans have the same amount of refined carbohydrates and the same number of calories—200.

8. The Muenster's 11 grams of saturated fat beat the pistachios' 3 grams easily. In addition, the pistachios contain monounsaturated fat, a good fat, as well as 7 grams of fiber—and no cholesterol!

9. Choose the banana. While the cookies have refined carbohydrates and saturated fat, the banana has 3 grams of fiber, no saturated fat, no cholesterol and only 100 calories.

10. The two Tofutti Chocolate Fudge Treats together cost a mere 60 calories. The single Weight Watchers Chocolate Fudge Bar comes in at 110 calories—and those calories come mostly from added sugar. The Tofutti Treats have zero added sugar.

CHAPTER 4

Vegetables: More Is Good, Even More Is Even Better

Ever think you'd find a weight loss book that would recommend that you eat more? Well, more is precisely the message we're delivering when it comes to vegetables. This is the one food group of which we can say without hesitation or reservation that the more you eat, the greater the benefits to you for weight loss and for preventing or managing diabetes.

The reasons? Vegetables are rich in two of the Four Phenoms that help lower your calorie intake and can actually reverse the effects of diabetes risk factors. First, they're loaded with fiber, and as you'll recall from our discussion in Chapter 2, fiber gives you that full feeling. Result? You're satisfied sooner, on less food, and the feeling of satiety lasts longer, so you take in fewer calories altogether over a twenty-four-hour period. More food with fewer calories: it's a good deal. And the bottom line of that good deal is simple: weight loss. (To see the deal in action, check out the Picture Perfect food demonstrations on pages 66–73.)

Second, vegetables are packed with phytonutrients that protect our bodies against the kind of cell damage diabetes can cause. They do so by strengthening the health of the blood vessels and, by lowering cholesterol and decreasing blood pressure, improving the composition of the blood. Among the cell-damaging effects phytonutrients can fight are stroke and heart attack, kidney disease, nerve damage, vision problems and more. The bottom line is simple here, too: more power to fight the effects of the disease.

That's why vegetables are the base of the Beat Diabetes Pyramid. They're the foundation of the Beat Diabetes eating plan—the bedrock on which the plan is based, the wellspring of all the advantages to be gained from eating the Pyramid way and following its guidelines. And just as the base of a pyramid occupies the greatest volume, so also should vegetables be the food group you eat the most of.

What do you think of when you think of vegetables? To many of you who may have tried weight-loss initiatives in the past, the very word may conjure up images of unadorned celery stalks or the overcooked spinach you loathed as a kid. Nothing could be further from the reality.

Gold, purple, deep orange, brilliant red, bright yellow and every shade of green.

Leaves, flowers, bulbs, stems, roots.

Growing underground, on vines, as the buds of plants, as their roots.

The world of vegetables is a universe of colors, textures, origins and tastes. Vegetables can be as ordinary as the much-maligned but delightfully crispy iceberg lettuce or as exotic as what the British call aubergine and we call eggplant. We read of favorite vegetables in ancient texts—like radishes, enjoyed by the Romans—and we associate certain vegetables with specific places—okra from the American South, leeks from the Celtic countries. And some vegetables have traveled farther than we're likely to in a lifetime: the tomato, native to the Americas, has become almost the national vegetable of Italy, to which it was introduced only in the sixteenth century. Marinara sauce, anyone?

In their sumptuous variety, vegetables form a rainbow of health that can arc across our lives. Where weight loss and managing diabetes are concerned, they're a good thing. And you remember what the legendary Hollywood vixen Mae West said on that score: "Too much of a good thing is wonderful!"

So why do some people, especially those who are diabetic or trying to lose weight, still shrink from certain vegetables that they suppose are fattening or bad for sugar control? You know the ones we mean: peas, beets, carrots—all the vegetables that seem sweet to the taste or that are starchy in texture.

GLYCEMIC INDEX, GLYCEMIC LOAD, GLYCEMIC IMPACT: THE REAL SKINNY

One reason may be all the talk about glycemic index—promoted by some researchers as measures of the effects of carbohydrates on blood sugar levels. The glycemic index number reflects how quickly sugars are absorbed into the bloodstream and raise the blood sugar level. The higher the glycemic index number, the more quickly the carbohydrates are absorbed and the faster the blood sugar level rises. Obviously, this is a very important concept for people suffering from diabetes or trying to lose weight, many of whom will aim to avoid vegetables with a fairly high glycemic index—for all practical purposes, anything over 50. That would include beets, with a glycemic index of 64, winter squash at 75, even carrots at 47—the sweet and starchy kinds of vegetables.

But there's an additional factor that needs to be taken into consideration: glycemic load. Glycemic load refines the glycemic index calculus by taking into account the amount of carbohydrates in an average serving of the particular food. In fact, when you factor in that refinement, you get a more accurate—and quite different—measure: beets have a glycemic load measurement of 5, carrots come in at 3 and winter squash's glycemic load is 3 as well.

Unfortunately, the idea of carrying around a chart of glycemic index and/or glycemic load numbers and basing your food choices on these measures can be burdensome for a lot of people, who may well decide that vegetables simply aren't worth the trouble.

Moreover, the fact is that a lot of different factors affect the speed with which a food's carbohydrate content will be absorbed into the bloodstream. Even such factors as how ripe the food is, how and when it was processed, how and for how long it's been stored, how it was cooked, even the particular variety of the food—green cabbage or red cabbage, for example—may affect the absorption rate.

It therefore makes much more sense to talk about *glycemic impact* rather than about the narrowly defined glycemic index and the only slightly more precise glycemic load. While glycemic index and glycemic load focus on one food in isolation, glycemic impact takes into consideration all the factors in your diet in general that affect how quickly sugars are absorbed in your bloodstream.

After all, you rarely eat a single food in isolation; rather, your meal consists of protein, fat, fiber, even acid—from the lemon juice or vinegar in your salad dressing, for example—and all these can affect how fast sugar enters into the blood. The balsamic vinegar on your salad of raw carrots and sweet peppers, to take just one delicious instance, helps to slow the rate at which your stomach empties, thereby slowing the rate at which glucose enters your bloodstream. So it simply doesn't work to take into account just the glycemic index number of the carrots or peppers onto which the balsamic vinegar is tossed. You've got to look at the total picture and assess the overall impact instead.

The beauty of the Beat Diabetes Pyramid is that it looks at the total picture; it assesses the overall impact of all the factors in your diet—the total glycemic impact as well as all the health impacts. In doing so, there's just no question that vegetables as a group remain the single most powerful weapon there is for achieving and maintaining weight loss and for beating diabetes. Yes, we'll have some important things to say about such starchy vegetables as potatoes and corn when we get to Chapter 6, but that these foods should be avoided is simply not true.

It's worth repeating: for weight loss and beating diabetes, where vegetables are concerned, more is good, and even more is even better.

GETTING TO MORE: PRACTICAL STEPS

Okay, how can you increase your intake of vegetables without feeling like you're swallowing something because your mother said there will be no dessert if you don't? Eat two salads instead of one? Force yourself to eat yet one more stalk of broccoli?

Well, that's one way to do it. But we have a couple of better suggestions.

Suggestion 1: Extend the Variety of Vegetables in Your Diet

Stop thinking of vegetables as just greens and as just raw, and start thinking out of the box. Roasted eggplant, marinated artichoke hearts, minestrone soup, grilled acorn squash, cauliflower casserole, pickled beets, sautéed spinach with garlic, Chinese stir-fry—all vegetable dishes.

Keep in mind also that you can get your vegetables in snacks, condiments, sauces, dips and toppings as well as entrées and at any time of day. While roasted eggplant or a Chinese stir-fry can be a meal unto itself, sautéed spinach is a great side dish, and artichoke hearts make an elegant hors d'oeuvre for the cocktail hour.

Remember, too, to get your vegetables in any form you can. Yes, in the summer, it's lovely to head for the nearest farmstand or local market for just-picked radishes, peppers, lettuces, beets and the like. But don't neglect the advanced technologies that have made it possible for us to have vegetables all year round by pulling a package out of the freezer or a can down from the pantry shelf. These days, the variety of vegetables on supermarket shelves and in supermarket freezers is pretty mind-boggling. Check it out.

EXTENDING YOUR VEGETABLE VARIETY

- Try grilled vegetables this summer. Marinate asparagus, eggplant, zucchini or other vegetables, or brush them with light barbecue sauce, and put 'em on the grill.

- You've heard of iceberg lettuce. What about romaine, Boston or butter lettuce, arugula (also called rocket), oak-leaf, Bibb, mâche or mesclun? Be adventurous.

- Vegetables are the cornerstone of good soups: carrot-ginger, curried pumpkin, squash, gazpacho, borscht, cucumber, tomato, minestrone.

- Stir-fry any combination of vegetables in hoisin sauce: cauliflower, peppers, onions, broccoli, green beans. You'll have a gorgeous, healthful, diabetes-beating, weight-losing meal in less than ten minutes.

Suggestion 2: Make It Tasty!

If you think that cooking vegetables means putting them in a pot of water and boiling them till all the flavor and nutrients are completely gone, you've got another think coming. In culinary academies, students rise or fall on the succulence of their vegetable preparations: presentation, texture and above all taste.

The possibilities are endless. Take it from Chef Franklin: you can live a lifetime and not run out of different ways to prepare utterly scrumptious vegetable dishes. Given the extraordinary variety of entries in this group plus the many different ways to prepare, flavor and cook foods, you are sure to run out of time before you run out of ideas for yet another vegetable dish. So for the adventurous cooks among you—or for the would-be cooks out there—go for it! Let your imagination run wild, and make vegetables the primary arena for your culinary inventiveness.

But even if you have neither the talent nor the inclination to make vegetables your cooking laboratory, there are still some very simple things you can do to make eating more vegetables something you'll look forward to. And since the more appetizing you find a food, the more you want to eat it, taste is extremely important.

You'll read more about sauces and condiments in Chapter 7, but here's the basic point: any sauce, dressing or seasoning that is not sugary in taste (except if it's sweetened with a low-calorie sweetener) and that is low in saturated fats or trans fats is particularly appropriate for enhancing the taste of vegetables. In other words, a honey-based dressing or butter-, cream- or cheese-based sauces are not going to work. Such additions are off the mark in terms of both diabetes management and weight loss—and not just where vegetables are concerned.

What works? Something as simple as lemon juice or as complex as balsamic vinegar brings out the flavor of the vegetable even as it adds its own piquant taste. And don't forget the other plus of these seasonings where fighting diabetes is concerned—the acid they contain slows the rate at which glucose enters the bloodstream.

Serving the same dual purpose of highlighting the underlying taste while adding enriching flavor are all the sauces and relishes of the great Asian cuisines: soy sauce, teriyaki sauce, hoisin sauce, curry paste, black bean sauce, Thai peanut sauce, sesame sauce and more. Hot sauces from the world's cultures—salsa, Tabasco, Worcestershire, wasabi—also work wonderfully well, and don't forget plain old mustard and ketchup. Best of all, many condiments, sauces, dips, toppings and dressings are themselves vegetable sources—chutneys, mole, salsa, caponata, ratatouille, marinara, pesto, pickled vegetable relishes and more.

SALT CAN BE YOUR FRIEND!

Soups, pickled vegetables, soy sauce: all recommended as ways to get you to eat more vegetables. But you may be wondering, what about the salt in these foods? After all, doesn't salt cause you to retain water and increase blood pressure?

Not really.

Yes, sodium intake—that is, salt—is one of many factors that influence fluid balance in the body. Other factors include hormone levels, temperature, humidity and the other foods you may eat. As those factors combine, you might find you weigh 2 pounds more tomorrow than you did today—and 3 pounds less the following day, just based on normal fluid balance.

But neither your fluid balance nor your salt intake has anything to do with diabetes control or losing fat—which is what you want to lose if you're overweight or obese.

Yes, salt can be a major factor in blood pressure control, but other factors are even more important, and most important of all is a way of eating that includes plenty of fruit, vegetables, plant-based proteins and ample amounts of "good" fat. In other words: the Beat Diabetes Pyramid.

So when you have an eating plan that is great for lowering blood pressure, for diabetes control and for weight loss, it makes sense to enjoy its health-promoting foods as much as possible. To that end, some salt, either on its own or in sauces and condiments, may well be essential for you—and that makes salt your friend.

For example, if the idea of plain steamed vegetables leaves you cold, you're unlikely to eat this crucial food group frequently enough or in sufficient quantity to derive its substantial health or weight-loss benefits. But if you flavor the steamed vegetables with black bean sauce, Thai peanut sauce or whatever else strikes your fancy, you'll eat them with pleasure.

The bottom line on salt? Take in however much you need to enjoy eating the Pyramid way. Whatever the amount, it makes salt your very good friend.

BOTTOM LINE

In short, that's exactly what vegetables are: the bottom line of weight loss and beating diabetes, the bedrock of a lifelong program for getting and staying healthy and of course the bottom rung of the Beat Diabetes Pyramid. You cannot do better for yourself—for your health and for your future—than to make vegetables the foundation of your eating.

As we said at the top of this chapter, vegetables are good. More vegetables are better. And even more vegetables are even better than that.

PIZZA AND...

More food for fewer calories—that's the promise of the Beat Diabetes Pyramid, and it's a promise fulfilled in this pizza demonstration:

On the left, two slices of pizza—an average portion to most folks. And what do these two slices deliver besides taste? A whopping 900 calories to burden your waistline and your heart! Nothing else.

Check out the meal on the right. Pizza may be the jewel in the crown of this lavish meal, but it is set between two equally delicious dishes—a substantial bowl of thick minestrone soup filled with vegetables and an antipasto as only the Italians can make it, with greens, tomatoes,

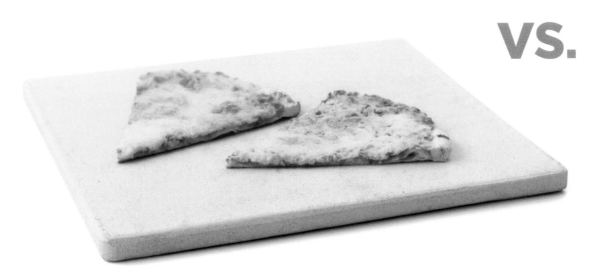

VS.

2 slices pizza
900 calories, 0 grams fiber

olives and marinated artichoke hearts. This is a full meal that will leave you feeling as satisfied as you are sated. And it's just 600 calories—far less than the two pizza slices to the left. Plus the 12 grams of fiber this meal provides will keep you feeling full, and that can keep you away from the table—or the fridge or the pantry—for hours and hours to come. It means fewer calories now—and fewer calories over the next twenty-four hours as well.

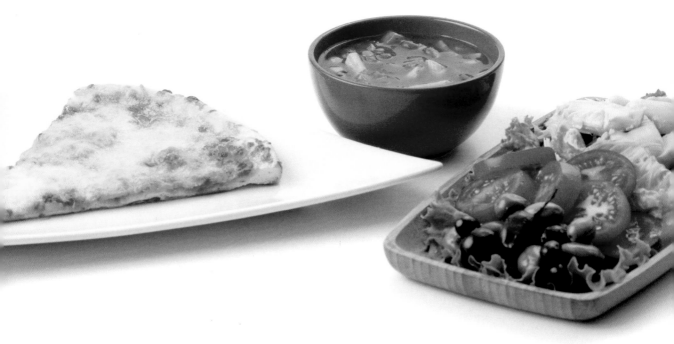

1 slice pizza	**450 calories**	**0 grams fiber**
1 bowl minestrone soup (1½ c.)	**110 calories**	**8 grams fiber**
Antipasto	**40 calories**	**4 grams fiber**
(greens, tomatoes, olives, marinated artichoke hearts)		

TOTAL **600** calories **12** grams fiber

SAILOR'S DELIGHT

Pasta with marinara sauce was the first thing sailors wanted to eat when they returned home to Naples after a tour on the high seas; that's where the name *marinara*—as in *marine*—comes from. But chances are that no sailor would be satisfied with that lonely-looking bowl of pasta on the left of the picture. Yet pasta and sauce together add a hefty 605 calories to the diet, while providing a mere 4 grams of fiber.

Appealing much more to the seafarer—or to anyone, for that matter—is the mouthwatering collection of foods to the right. The pasta with marinara sauce is there for the land-bound sailor. But in addition, there are broccoli rabe in garlic and olive oil, succulent herb-grilled tomato halves and sliced portobello mushrooms. All these dishes combined are a mere 355 calories, while the meal as a whole adds 11 grams of stomach-filling fiber to keep you feeling unhungry for a long time to come.

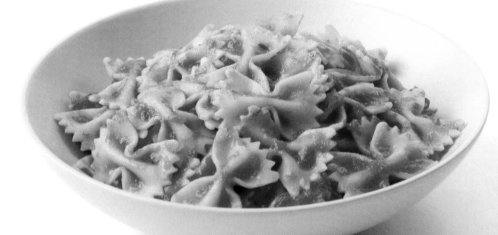

VS.

5 ounces pasta 525 **calories** 0 **grams fiber**
1 cup marinara sauce 80 **calories** 4 **grams fiber**

TOTAL 605 calories 4 grams fiber

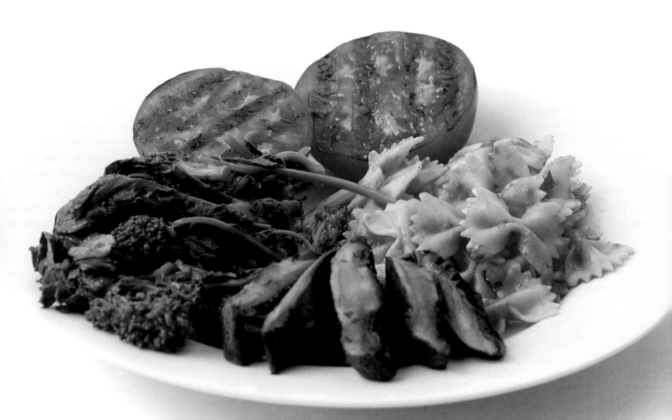

2 ounces pasta	**210 calories**	**0 grams fiber**
½ cup marinara sauce	**40 calories**	**2 grams fiber**
1 cup broccoli rabe with garlic and olive oil	**70 calories**	**4 grams fiber**
2 herb-grilled tomato halves	**20 calories**	**3 grams fiber**
Sliced portobello mushrooms	**15 calories**	**2 grams fiber**
TOTAL	**355 calories**	**11 grams fiber**

CURRIED PUMPKIN SOUP

½ cup chopped onion

½ cup chopped red or yellow bell pepper

½ cup chopped celery (including leaves)

1 tablespoon olive or canola oil

4 teaspoons curry powder

1 15-ounce can pumpkin

1 cup soy milk

1 cup water

1 tablespoon lemon juice

2–3 packets Splenda

1½ teaspoons salt

2 tablespoons chopped cilantro

1. **Combine the onion, peppers, celery and oil in a medium saucepan. Sauté over medium heat for 5 minutes, or until the vegetables are slightly tender.**

2. **Stir in curry powder and cook another minute.**

3. **Add pumpkin, soy milk, water, lemon juice, Splenda and salt.**

4. **Stir until well blended; cover pot and simmer over low heat for 15 minutes.**

5. **Pour into bowls, sprinkle with cilantro and serve.**

Yield: 5 servings

Each cup contains 85 calories, about 2½ grams of fat, 6 grams of fiber.

NOTE: **Fresh or frozen pumpkin or winter squash may be substituted for canned pumpkin.**

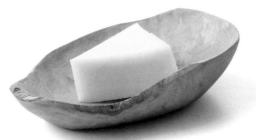

VS.

2-ounce chunk white cheddar cheese
230 **calories,** 19 **grams of fat**

Mutt and Jeff

Jeff is pictured on the left: a small chunk of white cheddar cheese. Enjoy this not particularly filling snack at your peril—especially if you are overweight or a diabetic or prediabetic. It contains 230 calories and 19 grams of fat, mainly saturated. Moreover, it doesn't contain a scintilla of fiber to give you that satisfied feeling.

Mutt is on the right: a curried pumpkin soup that is a delicious potpourri of vegetables—onions, peppers, celery and, of course, pumpkin. That makes it a powerhouse of phytonutrients such as beta-carotene and others, as well as a storehouse of fiber—6 grams per cup. All this for a mere 85 calories.

Try it yourself. This recipe makes about 5 cups, any one of which beats the cheese snack anytime—especially where weight loss and fighting diabetes are an issue.

1 cup Curried
Pumpkin Soup
85 calories
2½ grams of fat
6 grams of fiber

COCKTAIL HOUR

You can beat diabetes at any hour—even the cocktail hour. Take a look.

On the left is a typical pastry hors d'oeuvre: a couple of ounces of cheese straws that weigh in at 240 calories with 16 grams of saturated fat.

On the right a selection of vegetable and fish finger foods that altogether add up to a grand total of just 95 calories. But these cocktail offerings actually do you good, with 2 grams of "good" fat and 7 grams of fiber. Here's how these small canapés break down, showing you that even a small bite can make a big difference—for good or for ill:

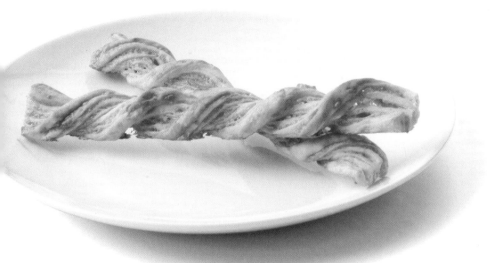

VS.

2 ounces cheese straws
240 calories, 16 grams fat,
0 grams fiber

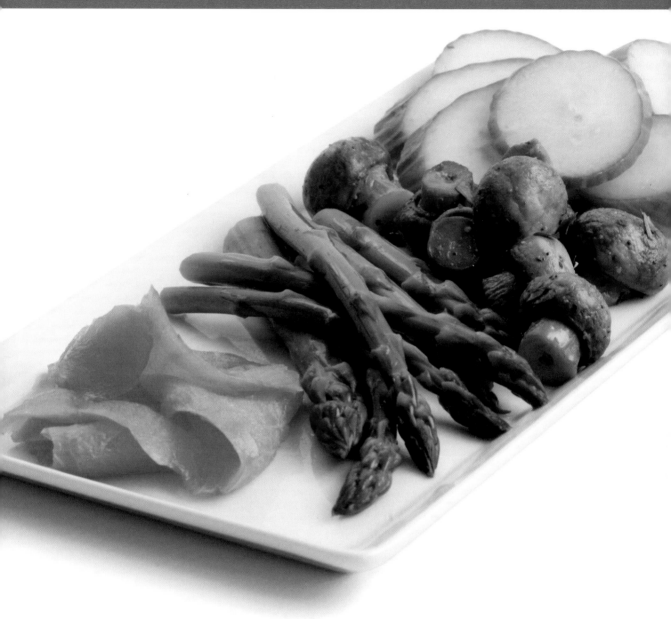

8 marinated mushrooms	20 calories	3 grams fiber	0 grams fat
7 pieces marinated asparagus	25 calories	3 grams fiber	0 grams fat
6 slices cucumber	5 calories	1 grams fiber	0 grams fat
1 ounce smoked salmon	45 calories	0 grams fiber	2 grams fat
TOTAL	95 calories	7 grams fiber	2 grams fat

CHAPTER 5

Protein: Expanding the Possibilities

The word *protein* comes from ancient Greek, and it means "being first." What that refers to is not a contest or a race; rather, it's about survival. Protein is the essential component of human cellular activity, playing a role in virtually every process of our body's functioning. We need protein to grow, to repair our cells, to keep our muscles and bones strong, to carry cell signals and prompt our immune responses, to execute all the biochemical reactions of metabolism.

Bottom line: we have to take in protein—or else.

For those trying to lose weight and prevent or manage diabetes, the best way to take in proteins is to focus on three food groups in particular, the three that form the protein rung of the Beat Diabetes Pyramid: legumes (beans, peas and lentils in all their variety), fish and soy foods.

Except for fish, those are probably not the foods that first leap to mind when you hear the word *protein.* Instead, you probably think of meat, poultry, eggs and dairy products. Certainly those are all protein foods. But where weight loss and diabetes are concerned, they are or should be a distant second choice as sources of protein, for along with the protein they undoubtedly deliver come a number of adverse effects that can undermine your attempts to lose weight and to prevent or manage the killer disease.

We'll go even further than that. The fact is that there are components in these sources of protein that may actually raise the risk of diabetes and its complications.

PROTEIN FOODS THAT DON'T BEAT DIABETES

What are the potential costs of these kinds of protein? They're high—and that's an assessment based on evidence that is both compelling and overwhelming.

Let's start with meat. Red meat such as steak, ribs and burgers has long been a staple of the American diet, and researchers have long been telling us it's a staple that can harm our health. The legendary Harvard study on nurses' health found, for example, that *for every serving of red meat you consume per day, you increase your risk of developing diabetes by 26 percent.*

The news is even worse for a serving of processed meat, which raises your risk of diabetes 38 percent, while a single serving of bacon increases the risk by a whopping 73 percent!

If you are already diabetic, the Harvard study found, red meat constitutes an *additional* health risk. That is, diabetics are already at least twice as likely as nondiabetics to suffer heart attack or stroke; a high intake of red meat exacerbates that unhappy equation. The Harvard nurses' study found that *consumption of red meat among diabetic women raised the risk of coronary heart disease by 50 percent over women who ate little or no red meat.*

Another staple of the American diet is eggs—the more or less standard breakfast in the local diner or coffee shop. For diabetics, however, eggs on a daily basis can exacerbate that already existing risk of heart disease. And studies are now showing that *an egg every day increases the risk—even the likelihood—of becoming diabetic;* specifically, the risk is increased by 58 percent in men and 77 percent in women.

That's not all eggs can do. In one study of more than 21,000 American physicians, *those who ate one or more eggs daily were 25 percent more likely to die of cardiovascular disease than those who ate one or fewer eggs weekly.*

As for dairy products, we can't avoid addressing the powerful evidence about the correlation between dairy consumption and diabetes. Study after study has suggested that cow's milk may trigger the production of antibodies that destroy insulin-producing cells. The correlation too often leads to type 1 diabetes in children. In a study of children with diabetes, 100 percent of them had high levels of one such antibody triggered by cow's milk protein.

But it isn't just children who may suffer. A British study on women and heart health found, among other conclusions, that milk-drinking women had lower insulin sensitivity and were more likely to have type 2 diabetes or metabolic syndrome.

Studies like these serve as a wake-up call for all of us concerned about the rise in the incidence of diabetes. They present what is by now a universally acknowledged truth: that a *diet high in red and processed meats, eggs and dairy products can increase every individual's risk of developing diabetes.*

Does that mean you should give up hamburgers forever and never again order eggs over easy at the diner downtown? Absolutely not. As we've said before, on the Beat Diabetes Pyramid, no food is forbidden. But we hope that with the increased awareness you'll gain in the pages of this chapter, you'll find yourself choosing more and more to avoid the costs of these kinds of protein in favor of the extraordinary gains from the three protein sources that constitute this rung of the Pyramid.

In short, for weight loss and preventing or managing diabetes, there are better ways to get your protein.

LOVELY LEGUMES

The first of the three is legumes—healthful, easy and a creative chef's delight. The names trip off the tongue like poetry: lima beans, navy beans, pinto beans, garbanzos, cannellini, black-eyed peas, fava beans, lentils. Legumes have been cultivated and eaten worldwide since the beginning of civilization. They embrace culinary possibilities that run from a plate of baked beans wolfed down at the barbecue to an elaborate French lentil soup flavored with tarragon and thyme and served with a vintage Bordeaux.

For our main focus—beating diabetes—**legumes are something of a perfect weapon: they are packed with fiber, loaded with phytonutrients that battle a range of health dangers, have no fat and no cholesterol and contain carbohydrates that are very slowly absorbed into the bloodstream and thus not an issue as far as blood sugar control is concerned.** And, of course, they deliver the goods—protein for all the body's functions.

They also offer a real plus when it comes to weight loss, which is so crucial to preventing or managing diabetes. That plus is the texture of these foods—their sheer density, which offers the same kind of satisfied feeling you get from eating starches, but, of course, without the starch. And since starch has its drawbacks when it comes to weight loss, as we'll explain in greater detail in the next chapter, legumes make an excellent substitute. Bottom line: they replace a food group that is not great for weight loss with one that is good for weight loss, while also offering the protein you need and the fiber and phytonutrients so important for overall health. It's a very, very good deal.

Texture is also the reason both professional and amateur chefs love legumes. Although beans, peas and lentils certainly offer a range of taste sensations, their utility as a culinary tool is their ability to take on the flavor of whatever they're cooked with. They can thus embody the collective experience of a combination of ingredients, serving as special vehicles of culinary creativity. So to all those weekend-warrior chefs and/or cooks hesitant to experiment, here's your chance. Create your own chilies, minestrone soups, lentil casseroles, three- or four- or eight-bean salads, falafel, hummus, refried beans, bean dips. Experiment with ingredients, accompaniments, condiments. Seize the legume opportunity and do yourself a favor constructing your own soups, salads and side dishes. You'll also be doing yourself—and your family—the favor of embracing a supremely healthful way to get the protein you all need.

FISH ISSUES

Fish is, of course, a great source of protein and a favorite culinary arena for chefs. From sushi to smoked salmon, from trout to tilapia, the variety of tastes, textures and cooking styles makes fish one of the core food groups.

Where fighting diabetes is concerned, the main benefit of fish is that it is low in saturated fat—versus meat, poultry or dairy—and can be an excellent source of omega-3 fatty acids.

Omega-3s deliver a range of health benefits and are powerful tools for controlling diabetes and its complications. Specifically, they help lower two key components of metabolic syndrome and major risk factors for the disease of diabetes: a high triglyceride count and high blood pressure. Indirectly, the omega-3s also affect weight loss; studies show that these fats actually help reduce insulin resistance, a major cause and/or complication of excess weight or obesity. If you're insulin-resistant, you're not regulating your blood sugar properly; this throws your carbohydrate and fat metabolic processes out of kilter, which in turn results in more weight gain—and can lead to or exacerbate diabetes. For several reasons, therefore, the omega-3s found in such richness in so many fish are great weapons for beating diabetes and maintaining a healthy weight—and thus constitute a good source of protein on the Beat Diabetes Pyramid.

But fish has issues. For one thing, it contains cholesterol. The cholesterol in fish, however, is not as much of a problem as the cholesterol in other animal foods because the latter—meat, poultry, dairy and eggs—contain saturated fat, and fish does not.

Another fish issue is in our ever-dirtier waterways—how pollution may be affecting fish. One certain effect has been an increase in the amount of mercury that fish absorb. As industrial mercury accumulates in water, it turns into methylmercury, which is a toxin that is particularly harmful to infants and young children. That is why the U.S. government has warned pregnant women about their intake of fish, asking them to limit their fish consumption to twice a week only and to meals of fish lower in mercury, such as shrimp, canned light tuna, salmon, pollock and catfish. That's a pretty potent advisory.

So are the advisories in more than thirty-five states about (PCBs), toxic and carcinogenic chemical compounds banned in 1979 but still accumulating in our waters. We don't take those concerns lightly.

But within the parameters of such concerns, we recommend fish as a protein source. With its high content of omega-3s and its relative lack of saturated fat, fish is a valuable alternative protein source, and it is certainly a preferable alternative to meat and chicken.

If you choose not to eat fish, you can get your omega-3s from flaxseeds or flax oil, from walnuts or in supplements made from flax and now from algae, which is where the fish get it.

MEATY MATTERS

Here are exact equivalent portions of red meat, chicken and fish. But portion size is where the equality stops. Have a look:

The differences are evident, and the bottom line is dramatic. The tuna steak comes in at almost half the calories of the beef steak. It offers one-fourth of the fat of red meat and about a third of the fat of the chicken. Just take a look at the fat visualizations—pats of butter for the steak and chicken, oil for the fish—to see the disparities. And where cholesterol is concerned, with its formidable consequences for health in general and diabetes in particular, there's simply no comparison in this comparison: the beef has nearly triple the tuna's cholesterol count, and the chicken has more than double.

7-ounce ribsteak

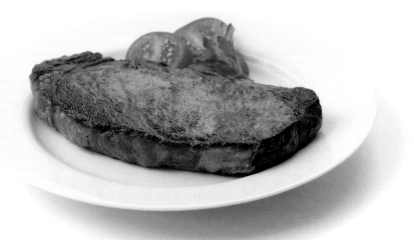

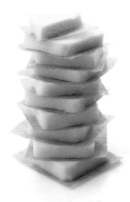

48 grams bad fat
= 9½ pats butter

**630 calories, 48 grams fat,
275 milligrams cholesterol**

7-ounce chicken
(leg and thigh with skin)

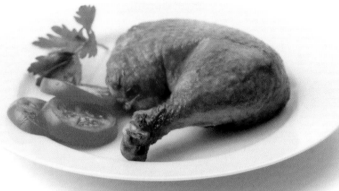

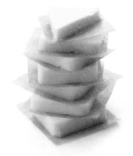

32 grams bad fat
= 6½ pats butter

506 calories, **32** grams fat,
240 milligrams cholesterol

7-ounce tuna steak

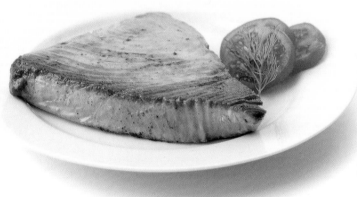

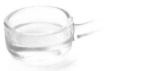

15 grams good fat
= 2½ teaspoons oil

344 calories, **12** grams fat,
85 milligrams cholesterol

The pats of butter you'll see in some of the food demos represent "bad fats"—the fats that are detrimental to general health, weight management and diabetes control.

The teaspoons of canola oil represent "good fats"—the fats that are essential for general health, weight management and diabetes control.

For more information on these fats and their food sources, see Chapter 7.

SINGULAR SOY

You've already read a good deal about soy protein in this book, and if it's beginning to look like we're stuck on soy, that's not far from the truth. There are two very powerful reasons for the emphasis on soy.

First, **soy is probably the single most potent weapon at your disposal for controlling diabetes and its complications and for helping you lose weight.** (It also decreases the risk of many cancers and helps prevent osteoporosis—just some of its additional benefits.) To repeat what we said back in Chapter 1, soy is a peerless diabetes fighter. Think of it: just by taking in this one food group with some regularity, you will not only defend your body against this killer disease but also actually prevent complications from the disease and even reverse its effects.

The main health benefits of soy where weight loss and diabetes are concerned? One more time:

1. Soy helps regulate glucose and insulin levels.
2. Soy proactively advances weight loss by burning body fat and instilling a sense of satiety.
3. Soy lowers the risk of cardiovascular disease or its severity.
4. Soy lowers the risk and slows the progression of kidney disease, a major complication of diabetes and one to which diabetics are particularly prone.

So soy as a diabetes fighter is the first reason we focus on it as much as we do.

SOY: IT'S WHAT'S FOR BREAKFAST, LUNCH, DINNER, SNACKS, APPETIZERS, PICNICS, ETC.

Soy-based products aren't just veggie burgers anymore. Here are just some of the myriad soy possibilities:

Breakfast: soy yogurt, soy shakes, breakfast sausage patties and links

Lunch: deli meats, veggie burgers, sloppy joes, veggie salads (chicken, turkey, egg)

Dinner: Thai- or teriyaki-flavored tofu cutlets eaten solo or for filling or toppings, pizza with veggie pepperoni, veggie Italian sausage and peppers, veggie ground beef in meat sauce or in chili or as taco filling

Snacks: roasted soybeans, edamame, soy crisps

Desserts: puddings and other soy-based desserts (see Chapters 2 and 8 for recipes)

Accompaniments: soy-based salad dressings and dips, soy "dairy" products (yogurt, cheese, sour cream), condiments like black soybeans with garlic and chilies, miso

---

The second reason for our emphasis on soy is that, despite its potency as a health weapon and its well-established place in some of the great cuisines of the world, most people in Western cultures are unaware of the range of soy foods available. Soy is the food industry's "newbie," and over the past few years, there has been a virtual explosion in the range and quality of the soy foods available. So part of our aim in this book is to raise your awareness of the many possibilities for making soy a part of your eating plan.

Basically, soy foods fall into two categories. The first is the traditional "pure" soy products known from the great cuisines of Asia: tofu, tempeh and miso. Steamed bean curd with mushroom sauce from Thailand, spicy tofu from China's Szechuan province or from Malaysia, the miso soup with which the Japanese start their days: these are some of the haute cuisine versions of soy served in restaurants—or in the homes of adventurous cooks, maybe like you.

The second category of soy foods is what we call "soy innovations." These are all the appetizers, snacks, breakfast or lunch or dinner foods, powders for shakes and puddings and meat alternatives you can find today on supermarket shelves everywhere. The veggie burger is the classic soy innovation, but today, the veggie burger is only the beginning. Take a look.

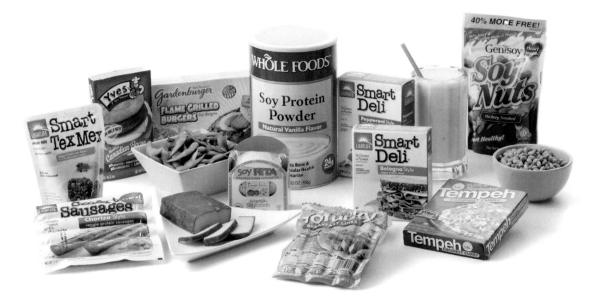

With these and many other soy innovations—we couldn't fit everything into a single photo!—the possible permutations for getting your soy are virtually endless. With pure soy, the beauty part for cooks is that the tofu or tempeh absorbs the flavors of whatever you're cooking it with. With soy innovations, all the taste mingling has already been done for you; all you have to do is serve. That doesn't mean, however, that soy innovations leave nothing to the creative culinary imagination; as you'll see in some of the recipes in this book, you can use soy innovations to devise a range of meals and snacks.

Try this ginger fruit yogurt for breakfast—and get not only protein but the added benefits of phytonutrients and fiber:

GINGER FRUIT YOGURT

1 6-ounce container plain soy yogurt

½ cup diced fruit (apples, bananas, peaches, strawberries, etc.)

2-3 packets Splenda

½ teaspoon vanilla extract

½ teaspoon ground ginger

Stir ingredients together in a mixing bowl till well blended. Refrigerate at least 30 minutes before serving.

Yield: one 180-calorie serving.

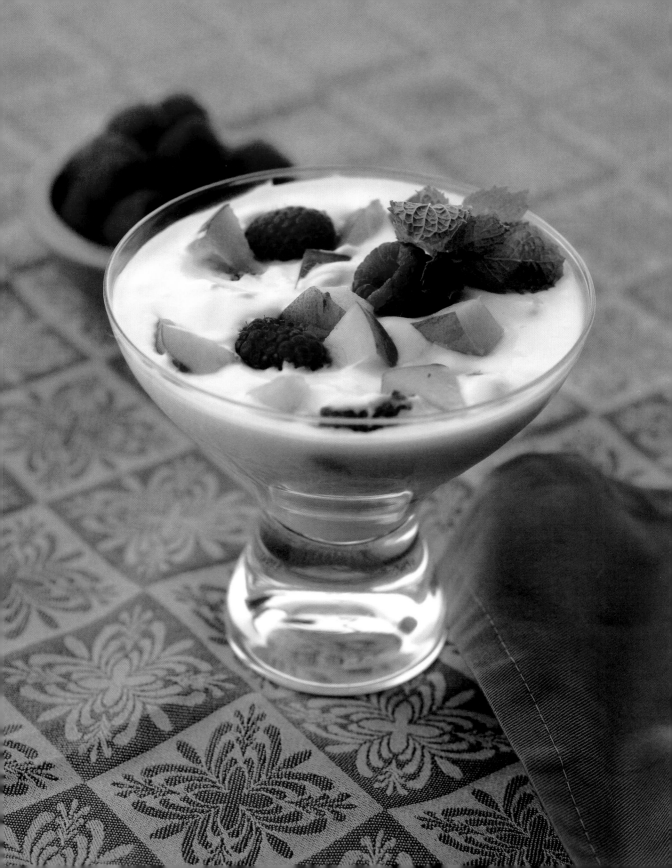

NO BALONEY

Want deli for lunch? Here are a few choices:

3 ounces beef-and-pork bologna

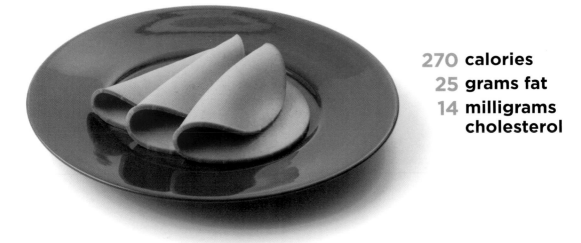

270 **calories**
25 **grams fat**
14 **milligrams cholesterol**

3 ounces turkey bologna

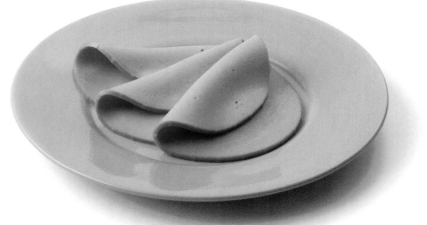

180 **calories**
15 **grams fat**
120 **milligrams cholesterol**

The traditional beef-and-pork bologna costs you 270 calories and burdens your body with substantial saturated fat and cholesterol. The turkey bologna slices off some numbers but still leaves you with substantial amounts of calories, fat and cholesterol.

3 ounces "veggie" bologna

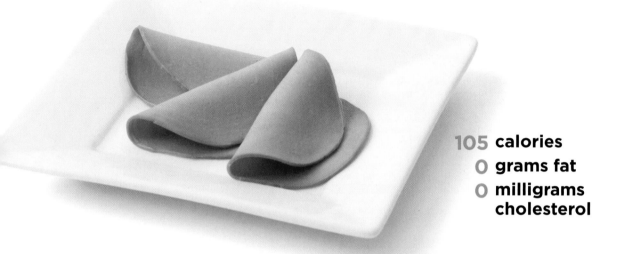

105 calories
0 grams fat
0 milligrams cholesterol

Behold now the veggie or soy-based bologna: a mere 105 calories—and no fat or cholesterol whatsoever.

Same portion sizes, same tastes, wildly different health impacts—and that's no baloney.

This crescendo of possibilities for taking in soy makes it downright easy to get the extraordinary benefits this food offers for weight loss and fighting diabetes, as well as for so many other health issues. As a protein source, it not only lacks the negatives of meat, poultry, eggs and dairy, but it can actually counteract those negatives *and* add positive advantages.

For example, there's no more deadly complication of diabetes than cardiovascular disease; it is, as we know, the number one killer disease of our time. Yet there are components in meat, poultry, eggs and dairy foods that can actually increase the risk of heart disease and stroke. Eat a hamburger, and its content of saturated fat and cholesterol raises your risk of cardiovascular problems and ups the chances that the problems will be severe.

A soy-based veggie burger, by contrast, not only counteracts those effects, but it also proactively strengthens your cardiovascular system. Here's what the tiny soybean does for your heart health: it strengthens your blood vessels, improves the composition of your blood by lowering the amount of total and LDL cholesterol, prevents the oxidation of LDL cholesterol, lowers your triglyceride count, regulates your blood sugar and helps you lose weight. That's a lot of bang for the buck, and with soy innovations, you can enjoy those benefits easily and in varied ways.

A BETTER BURGER

For further evidence that soy-based foods are the preferable protein alternative to meat or poultry, here it is by the numbers.

5-ounce beef burger

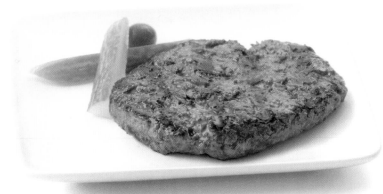

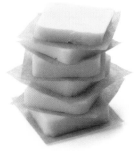

26 grams bad fat
= 6 pats butter

**308 calories, 26 grams fat,
130 milligrams cholesterol, 0 grams fiber**

5-ounce turkey burger

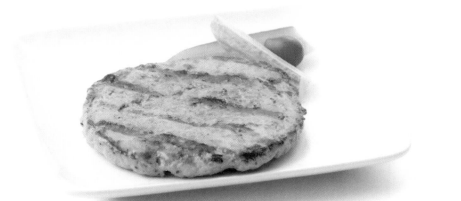

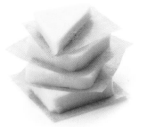

14 grams bad fat
= 3½ pats butter

**230 calories, 14 grams fat,
116 milligrams cholesterol, 0 grams fiber**

5-ounce veggie burgers

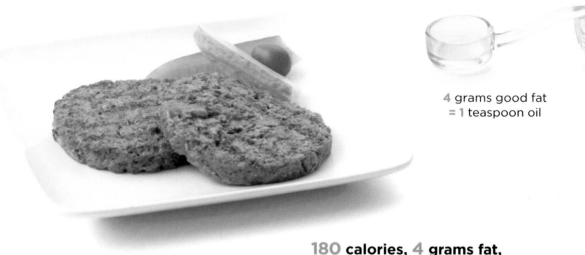

4 grams good fat
= 1 teaspoon oil

**180 calories, 4 grams fat,
0 milligrams cholesterol, 8 grams fiber**

Again, we're not asking you to exclude or limit other protein sources. But it's important for you to know why meat, poultry, eggs and dairy are not on the Beat Diabetes Pyramid, and it's equally important for you to be aware of the rich and tasty protein possibilities the Pyramid offers.

HOW MUCH?

So how much legumes, fish and soy should you take in to get the protein your body absolutely requires and fight diabetes at the same time?

As we have throughout this book, we offer no specific measure of "correctness"; our mantra, as always, is to eat when hungry and stop eating when satisfied.

But for the three food groups on the protein rung of the Beat Diabetes Pyramid, we're happy to suggest that "satisfied" should be interpreted as generously as possible. In other words, if you think you'd like one more veggie meatball or yet another handful of roasted soy nuts, don't hesitate. Where these sources of protein are concerned, there's no problem making sure your appetite and taste buds are as satisfied as possible.

CHAPTER 6

Starches

Remember high-school biology? In the segment on photosynthesis, we all learned how plants use the energy they get from sunlight to produce glucose, which is stored in the form of starch. That makes starchy foods great energy sources for humans. In fact, starch is more or less the most basic carbohydrate in the human diet—a source of quick, sustained energy. Rice, wheat, corn, barley, quinoa, oats, millet and potatoes are eaten around the world, ingredients of the most basic foods of every culture, from Mediterranean flatbread and Mexican tortillas to a coarse rye bread or a slender French baguette, Moroccan couscous to Asian rice.

For our purposes—losing weight and preventing or managing diabetes—**the starchy foods on the Beat Diabetes Pyramid offer the gift of fiber,** an important benefit, and one of the Four Phenoms for beating the killer disease. You remember the reasons. First of all, fiber is filling—a big plus for weight loss. But as you recall from Chapter 1, fiber offers even more diabetes-fighting power. It helps maintain insulin levels by slowing the absorption of sugar into the bloodstream. It lowers blood pressure and reduces total and LDL cholesterol and triglyceride counts, thus in turn reducing the risk of heart disease, a key complication of the disease.

In fact, as we also said back in Chapter 1, fiber is the one nutrient in the fight against diabetes to which we can actually assign a recommended daily amount to consume: at least 25 to 30 grams—easy to get if you follow the Pyramid guidelines and get your fiber from a range of sources, enjoying a range of tastes and textures in a varied eating plan.

The reason starches occupy a smaller rung than vegetables or the fiber-filled legumes of the protein rung is because they are not the most calorically economical way to get fiber. For the same amount of fiber as you would get in green beans, for example, a starch can cost you substantially more in calorie count. Or take a look at the demonstration featuring cauliflower on the next page.

CALORIE ECONOMICS

The whole-grain brown rice on the Beat Diabetes Pyramid offers more fiber for the same number of calories as the white rice, which, as a refined grain product, does not make it onto our Beat Diabetes Pyramid at all. But look at the vegetable, cauliflower; it achieves the same high fiber content at a much lower calorie count than even the whole-grain starch. That's why starches are afforded a smaller rung on the Pyramid than vegetables.

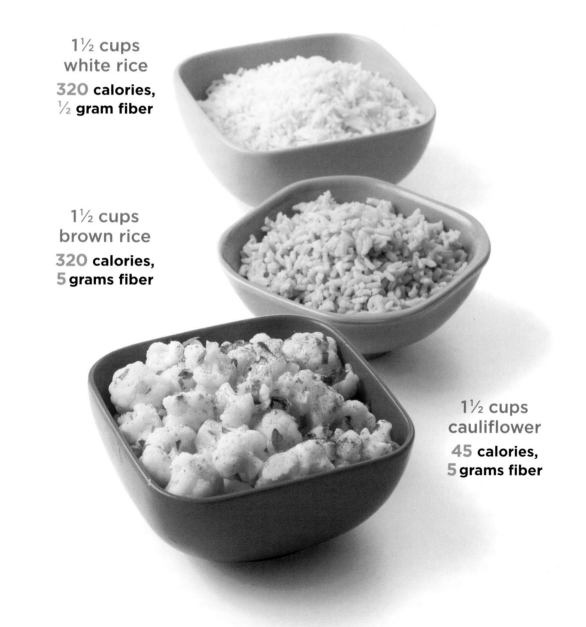

1½ cups white rice

320 calories, ½ gram fiber

1½ cups brown rice

320 calories, 5 grams fiber

1½ cups cauliflower

45 calories, 5 grams fiber

Nevertheless, in a varied diet—and especially in their role as sideshow to the main courses of vegetable and protein—starches serve as excellent delivery mechanisms for getting part of your recommended daily hit of fiber and all its benefits.

And the best way to get the fiber benefit from starchy foods is through whole-grain products, light and high-fiber breads and such starchy vegetables as corn and sweet potatoes.

WHAT'S WHOLE ABOUT WHOLE GRAIN?

Why whole-grain products? The answer is simple: they're the ones with the nutrients. In order to make the foods that derive from grains, the grains are put through a refining process that strips off the germ of the grain and its outer bran layer, leaving only the starchy part. Yet it is precisely in the germ and bran that the nutrients are found: B-complex vitamins, vitamin E and the fiber so important to weight loss and fighting diabetes. There is so little nutrition left in refined grain products that farmers report that even bugs die when trying to sustain themselves on it in silos.

The whole-grain products, therefore—brown rice rather than white, whole-grain pasta and polenta, whole-grain cereals and breads—are thus better for your health in general, and if you're trying to lose weight and prevent or manage diabetes, their fiber content provides an extra benefit. So as you shop for grain products in the market—cereals, pastas, rice, bread—make sure you look for the whole-grain version (see the sidebar to know how to be sure). And in your favorite restaurant, make a point of stressing that whole-grain products are what you prefer to order.

THE HOLE IN WHOLE GRAIN

Whole grains! Harvest wheat! Organic! Natural! Healthy!

So proclaim the marketing banners sprawled across bread packages. But look closely. Whatever the size of the print, does the package really say "whole grain," or does it just "contain" whole grains or come "with" whole grain?

There was a time when "whole grain" meant just that. But now, consumers need to beware the circumlocutions of marketing. Here's the reality: unless the package clearly states "100 percent whole grain," or unless a whole grain is the very first item listed in the ingredients list, it isn't whole grain.

OTHER BREADS

Still, don't feel that whole grain is the only bread you can eat when you're trying to lose weight or fight diabetes. There are other options. You'll find them in supermarkets under a range of labels: light breads, high-fiber breads and low-carb breads. Check out the photograph below to see something of the variety of these breads available.

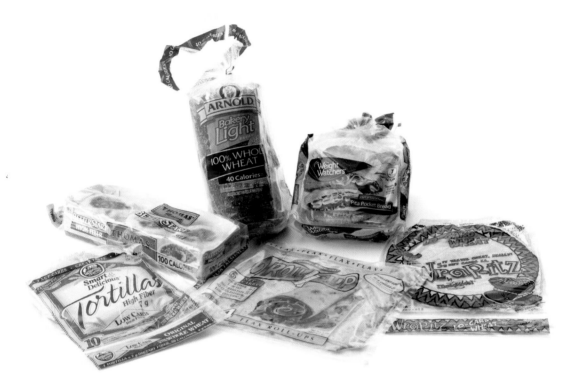

Light breads have fewer calories than both whole-grain and refined bread—some 40 or 45 calories per slice versus 80 or 100—but they contain the same amount of fiber as whole grain and sometimes even more. The reason? To get the calories down, the manufacturers of these breads use fiber ingredients such as wheat bran, thus raising the fiber content while lowering the caloric impact.

CEREALS

Cereal presents another dilemma altogether—namely, the sheer number of choices. Walk down the cereal aisle of any supermarket today, and you will grow dizzy from the number and variety of breakfast possibilities. It can be downright confusing.

As with bread packages, beware the marketing slogans, and read the fine print. The package of a particular cereal may scream that it contains soy protein, omega-3s or fiber, promising that you can get the health-giving benefits of these components early and easily with just a quick bowl of the cereal. Turn the package around, however, to check the ingredients list, and you may find that in addition to protein, omega-3s and fiber, the cereal also contains a virtual truckload of sugar.

Here are three different types of cereal—refined, whole grain, and high fiber, including some of the very best-known brands. Each type has approximately the same number of calories in a cup—around 100 to 140. But note the stunning difference in fiber content.

The refined cereals—the Kellogg's Corn Flakes and Rice Krispies that have fed generations of Americans—provide not quite a single gram of fiber in a cup.

Whole-grain cereals such as Wheaties and Cheerios do considerably better—3 to 4 grams. But their fiber content pales by comparison to the knockout fiber content of the high-fiber cereals such as Fiber One and All-Bran Extra Fiber. The latter provide a full day's recommended fiber allotment in a single cup of breakfast cereal. That makes these cereals a real fiber bargain.

So how can you get past the slogans and taglines, not to mention the confusion, and choose a good cereal—one that will offer the fiber benefits you're looking for without the infusion of sugar that afflicts so many commercial cereals? Here's a simple guideline: **look for a cereal that contains at least 3 grams of fiber per serving and no more than 6 grams of sugar per serving.** Whatever else it may contain, if the cereal follows those two guidelines, it's a good cereal for helping you lose weight and fight diabetes.

STARCHY VEGETABLES

If this were a contest, corn and sweet potatoes would beat out even whole-grain starches in terms of weight control and fighting diabetes. Certainly, these starchy vegetables have fewer calories and far more fiber than refined products; plus, they add the bonus of phytonutrients.

And while whole-grain and high-fiber breads are also great sources of fiber and phytonutrients, they're less economical calorically than the vegetables.

But of course, this is not a contest. Instead, all three kinds of foods—whole grains, light or high-fiber or low-carb breads and starchy vegetables—are good ways for those trying to lose weight and fight diabetes to get their fiber.

CEREALS—ALL 1 CUP

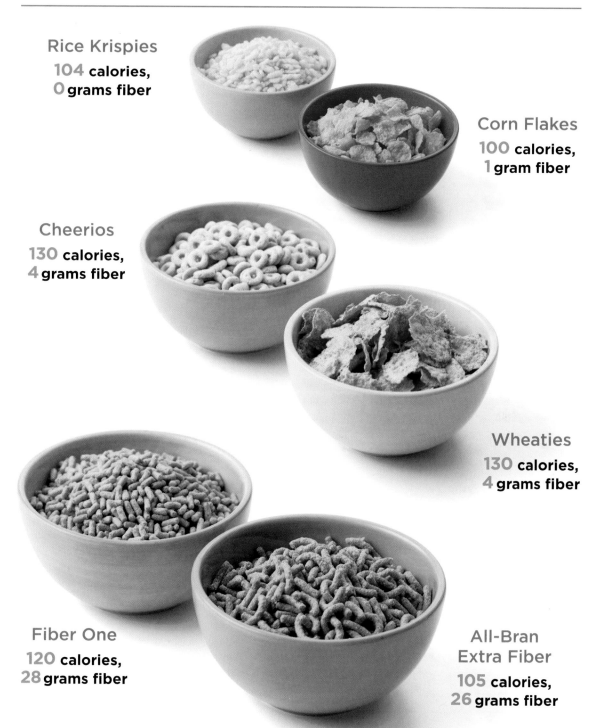

Rice Krispies
104 calories,
0 grams fiber

Corn Flakes
100 calories,
1 gram fiber

Cheerios
130 calories,
4 grams fiber

Wheaties
130 calories,
4 grams fiber

Fiber One
120 calories,
28 grams fiber

All-Bran Extra Fiber
105 calories,
26 grams fiber

THE STARCHY VEGETABLE ADVANTAGE

Here's another look at the fiber advantage vegetables provide over refined starches. This portion of rice costs 440 calories and delivers less than 1 gram of fiber. Contrast it with this vegetable plate containing corn and baked sweet potato. The corn comes in at 90 calories with 3 grams of fiber, the potato at 100 calories with 4 grams of fiber. Total for the veggie plate: 190 calories, less than half of what the rice contains, and a full 7 grams of fiber.

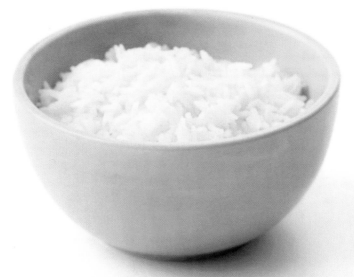

2 cups of white rice
440 calories,
>1 gram fiber

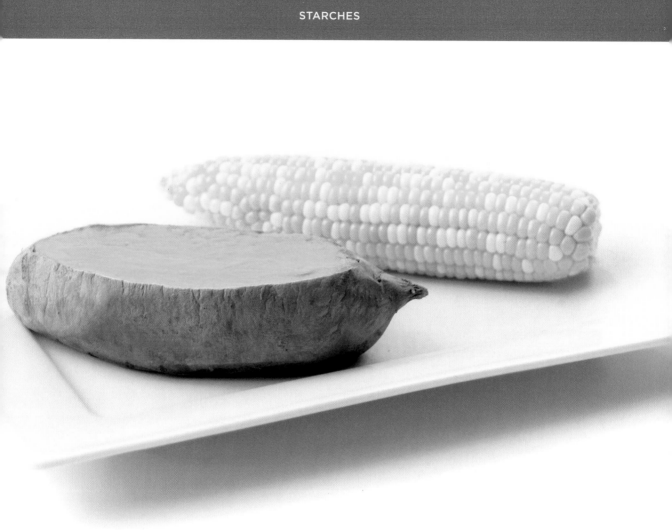

Ear of corn   90 **calories** 3 **grams fiber**
Baked sweet potato 100 **calories** 4 **grams fiber**

TOTAL **190** calories **7** grams fiber

BOTTOM LINE

But here's the last word on the starches in the Beat Diabetes Pyramid: don't rely on them as your sole or even main source of fiber. Instead, make them side dishes or accompaniments in a varied diet.

Above all, make sure your eating plan contains proportionally more of the two base rungs of the Pyramid—vegetables and protein—than of starches.

CHAPTER 7

Fats and Oils

The difference is as clear as day and night, heaven and hell, Red Sox and Yankees.

On one side are the "bad" fats: saturated fats and trans fats. Saturated fats—often solid at room temperature—are the fats found in animal foods: meat, poultry, dairy and eggs. To be fair, some vegetable products—palm oil, for example—also contain saturated fats. These fats raise total and LDL cholesterol levels, which is harmful to heart health, and burden insulin receptors, which raises the risk of diabetes.

Trans fats, which start as liquids and are solidified through the process of hydrogenation, also raise LDL cholesterol levels. In addition, they lower the level of HDL cholesterol, decrease the body's ability to burn fat and raise the levels of C-reactive protein—a marker for inflammation. Trans fats extend the shelf life of many commercial food products; they're

THE HEALTH STUDY PENDULUM

For a long time, we were told butter, a saturated fat, was bad for us, so we should all put margarine on our bread—a vegetable fat considered a healthy substitute.

Enter trans fats! The popular thinking changed again. Since many margarines are high in trans fats, we would all be better off going back to butter.

But the numbers tell a different story. In general, margarine contains 11 percent saturated fat and 1 percent trans fat, while butter contains 40 percent saturated fat and 5 percent trans fat. So even the worst of margarines is probably not as harmful as butter—especially if you're trying to lose weight or fight diabetes.

Recently, many margarine manufacturers, eager to be able to proclaim "no trans fat" on their packaging, have substituted palm oil for the hydrogenated oil in the margarine. True, palm oil has no trans fat, but it's very high in saturated fat.

Margarine guidelines? Look for products listing vegetable oil—preferably canola or olive— as their first ingredient. Also, a soft tub margarine rather than a solid stick is usually a better bet. Moreover, several light margarines on the market offer considerably fewer calories than regular margarine. In cooking, olive oil or canola oil is always preferable to any margarine.

And assume that the pendulum won't swing back.

found in vegetable shortenings and margarines, crackers, cookies, processed pastries, snack foods and—famously—such fried foods as french fries. And as we've noted, 25 percent of the vegetables eaten in the United States are french fries!

While cholesterol is not a fat, it plays on the Bad Fats team. That is because it often occurs together with fat in all animal products, and although this dietary cholesterol does not raise blood cholesterol as much as do saturated and trans fats, it raises it somewhat. Moreover, it works synergistically with saturated fat; that is, a food that has both saturated fat and cholesterol will raise blood cholesterol to a greater degree and with more impact than a food that does not. Shrimp, for example, has virtually no fat, but it does have cholesterol. Salmon, by contrast, has both cholesterol and fat, but not saturated fat. Neither will have nearly as much of an impact on blood cholesterol as a steak, a cheese omelet or a side order of bacon.

On the other side of the line is Team Good Fats, comprising monounsaturated and polyunsaturated fats and omega-3 fatty acids. These good fats do exactly the opposite of what the bad fats do—and more. **Healthful fats lower cholesterol and may decrease insulin resistance. In addition, the omega-3s lower triglycerides, raise HDL cholesterol, lower blood pressure and can help prevent blood clotting. They boost the level of leptin, the hormone that helps regulate appetite and metabolism, and they stimulate the body's fat-burning mechanism. They can even help keep glucose intolerance from turning into full-blown type 2 diabetes.**

THE CHALLENGE

All fats, good and bad, represent a very concentrated source of calories—approximately 100 to 125 calories per tablespoon. That doesn't mean you should avoid the good fats. The main reason fats and oils occupy such a small rung of the Beat Diabetes Pyramid is not their calorie count; it's because in general, fats and oils represent a smaller portion of the overall diet than other foods. Their primary role is really to flavor foods and enhance their appeal.

Fat is crucial to the functioning of the body—especially for skin, hair, blood and brain—and, as you remember from Chapter 1, it offers substantive benefits for weight loss and for beating diabetes. So we must take in fats; in fact, certain fatty acids are labeled essential because they are not made by the body and must therefore be obtained through food.

The challenge, therefore, is to balance your intake of fats so you get enough of the weight loss and diabetes-fighting benefits while avoiding a calorie intake that could jeopardize those very benefits.

Fortunately, by following the guidelines of the Beat Diabetes Pyramid, you should be able easily to achieve the right balance.

How? Guideline 1

Note the team players in the fats and oils rung of the Pyramid:

- Canola, flax and olive oils
- All nuts and seeds and their butters and oils
- Olives
- Avocado

All of these contain good fats. Basically, we're talking about oils for cooking and for use in dressings and dips; about snack foods—nuts, seeds, olives; and about the basis of guacamole, avocado, also a salad food.

A NUTTY REPLACEMENT

A transatlantic study on almonds and cholesterol found not only that almonds helped maintain a healthy cholesterol level without weight gain but also that study participants found the nuts sufficiently filling that they used them to replace other foods. Over a period of ten weeks, study participants neither gained weight nor increased their body fat—nor did they increase the amount of food they were eating.

In addition, levels of vitamin E and magnesium were up in the study participants, a direct effect of the intake of almonds.

How Much? Guideline 2

The fact is that as a general rule, we usually don't eat a huge volume of fat or oil. In that respect, the foods on the fats and oils rung are typical; none of them represents anything like high-volume eating. We might use a tablespoon or two of the oils at any one time, munch a handful of nuts, seeds or olives and enjoy avocado as an appetizer, side dish or light lunch. But that's about it. The amount of these fats we take in tends to be basically modest relative to other food groups.

And that's pretty much all that's needed to get the benefits of the Beat Diabetes fats and oils. A good amount of omega-3s per day, for example, would be from 1 to 3 grams—especially if you have or are at risk for high blood pressure or high triglycerides. Where can you find 3 grams of omega-3s? A single tablespoon of flaxseeds provides just that amount; sprinkle it on a salad, fruit or pretty much anything else. One tablespoon of flax oil, by contrast, contains 7 grams of omega-3s, so a single teaspoon of flax oil on your salad would do the trick.

In fact, try this quick and easy recipe for sesame-flax dressing—worthy of a Good Fat award.

SESAME-FLAX DRESSING

1. Put the ingredients together in a jar.

2. Refrigerate, then shake again before using.

The recipe makes ten 2-tablespoon servings at 90 calories per serving.

¼ cup toasted sesame oil	¼ cup prepared mustard
¼ cup flax oil	2 packets of Splenda
¼ cup vinegar	¼–½ teaspoon salt
¼ cup water	Pepper to taste.

Don't forget that every tablespoon of oil, no matter what kind, costs 100 to 125 calories. So while you might be using olive oil, for example, to replace a bad fat, the fact that it is a good fat should not be license to slather it extravagantly over everything.

OLIVE OIL PREMIUM

It's called squalene, and a study has shown that it lowers LDL cholesterol. Patients participating in the study took squalene supplements for five months and enjoyed a 22 percent decline in their LDL cholesterol count. But olive oil contains squalene naturally, so just by substituting it for butter, you may be lowering your bad cholesterol.

Another study suggests that extra-virgin olive oil may even go one step further than refined olive oil, protecting against LDL cholesterol oxidation.

This cholesterol-lowering power makes olive oil a highly rewarding good fat.

How to split the difference? Follow the mantra used throughout this book: let your appetite and sense of satiety be your guide. Where the oils for cooking are concerned, use the amount you need to enhance the flavor of other foods on the Pyramid; in a salad or dressing, use enough to satisfy your taste. Enjoy that handful of nuts, seeds or olives, and if one avocado half isn't enough, by all means have the other.

Here's the bottom line: an eating plan that contains fairly liberal amounts of the good fats but is restricted in refined carbohydrates is good for both diabetes control and weight loss. The Beat Diabetes Pyramid is such an eating plan, so where the good fats are concerned, be a liberal, not a conservative.

DIPS AND DRESSINGS

Here are examples of appetizer dips, salad dressings and side dishes, lined up as bad fats versus good. Check out the calorie differences in these particular dips and dressings—with no sacrifice of taste.

Bad Fats

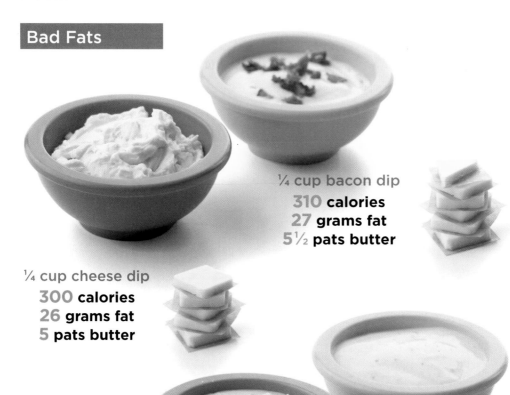

¼ cup bacon dip
310 calories
27 grams fat
5½ pats butter

¼ cup cheese dip
300 calories
26 grams fat
5 pats butter

¼ cup ranch dressing
344 calories
18 grams fat
3½ pats butter

¼ cup blue cheese dressing
320 calories
28 grams fat
5½ pats butter

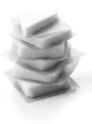

Good Fats

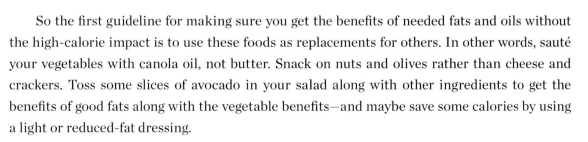

¼ cup hummus
104 calories
6 grams fat
1 teaspoon oil

¼ cup guacamole
110 calories
10 grams fat
2 teaspoons oil

¼ cup creamy Italian
dressing
216 calories
22 grams fat
4½ teaspoons oil

¼ cup Dijon
vinaigrette
228 calories
23 grams fat
4½ teaspoons oil

So the first guideline for making sure you get the benefits of needed fats and oils without the high-calorie impact is to use these foods as replacements for others. In other words, sauté your vegetables with canola oil, not butter. Snack on nuts and olives rather than cheese and crackers. Toss some slices of avocado in your salad along with other ingredients to get the benefits of good fats along with the vegetable benefits—and maybe save some calories by using a light or reduced-fat dressing.

GOOD FAT/BAD FAT

Here's the good fat vs. bad fat story in a nutshell—to be specific, a peanut shell:

On the left, 2 tablespoons of butter. It's not a huge amount, yet the butter contains 220 calories and 24 grams of fat—indicated as 5 pats of butter. And butter is mainly saturated fat; it raises your cholesterol and has no redeeming health benefits.

On the right, an equivalent amount of peanut butter: 2 tablespoons. The peanut butter contains fewer calories (190) and less fat (16 grams, represented as 3 teaspoons of oil) than the butter. But this fat is mainly monounsaturated, so it may actually lower your cholesterol. Moreover, it contains such vitamin and mineral nutrients as vitamin E, niacin, phosphorus and magnesium.

End of story.

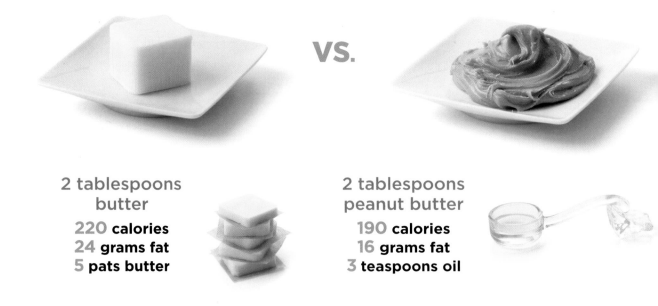

VS.

2 tablespoons
butter

220 calories
24 grams fat
5 pats butter

2 tablespoons
peanut butter

190 calories
16 grams fat
3 teaspoons oil

CHAPTER 8

Sweets

On most food pyramids, the peak rung comes with what amounts to a warning sign: eat very little of these foods! That's why the top rung is so small. Proportionately, you're supposed to have only a small taste.

Not on the Beat Diabetes Pyramid. The sweets that made it onto the top rung here—fruit, no-added-sugar frozen fudge pops and ice pops, many no-added-sugar candies, other sugar-free desserts, even chocolate—all qualify as fighters for weight loss and against diabetes, and you can eat generous amounts of them.

In fact, the only reason these foods occupy such a small rung is that sweets tend to be a small part of eating in general. After all, the word *dessert* comes from a French verb meaning "to clear away the dishes," and sweets are indeed the incidental food—an elegant final flourish after the meal or a quick taste you crave in an afternoon snack. These aren't foods that take up a large space on the plate or carry out a large role in any eating plan.

But there's no denying that the so-called sweet tooth is a universal human characteristic. From time to time, everyone craves the rich pleasures of sweet tastes, and it would be foolish—and ineffectual—to deny that appetite or set limits on it.

And as the sweets at the top of the Beat Diabetes Pyramid prove, you don't have to. Like all the foods on the Pyramid, the sweets at the top are there for good reasons, should be eaten and should be enjoyed generously.

To many people, of course, the idea that diabetics or those trying to prevent diabetes should eat sweets sounds not just weird but downright heretical. After all, these people ask, *aren't sweets the very first group of foods diabetics are told to abandon? Not these sweets. There are sweets on the Beat Diabetes Pyramid that literally fight diabetes and its complications and help weight loss.* Others are there because they offer the promise of sweetness without some of the burdens that some sweet foods do indeed carry: bad fats, for example, or refined carbohydrates. The latter therefore satisfy the sweet tooth that every human has but do so in a completely neutral way. That's why they play an important role in any overall eating plan.

Let's take the sweets one at a time.

FRUITS

Like vegetables, fruits present a wide-ranging and multicolored variety of tastes and textures. And, like vegetables, to those seeking to lose weight and prevent or manage diabetes, they offer the powerful pluses of fiber and phytonutrients with a low calorie content.

What often makes people hesitate about fruit is that it contains sugar. And it is true enough that the sugar it contains is no different from the sugar in the richest-tasting candy bar or the most elaborate pastry. After all, sugar is sugar.

But the amount of sugar in fruit is far less than the amount in even a small portion of candy or pastry, as you'll see in the demonstrations that follow. And whereas the candy and pastry are made with refined carbohydrates and thus lack any nutritional value, the fruit is packed with the phytonutrients and fiber that help you lose weight and fight diabetes.

NO "GOOD" OR "BAD" FRUIT

Remember back in Chapter 4 when we talked about glycemic index and glycemic load vis-à-vis vegetables? You'll recall that the index measures how quickly the sugars in food enter the bloodstream, and that glycemic load refines that measure by factoring in the amount of carbohydrates in an average serving of the food. We concluded that what really makes sense is to take into consideration all the factors in the diet and thereby look at overall glycemic impact. The same is true of fruits.

For example, the glycemic index of watermelon is 72, a high measure that might put you off eating it. Its glycemic load is 4, which is low and would encourage you to eat it. But in addition, nutrients in the rest of the meal you've eaten or in the diet as a whole need to be taken into consideration to get a sense of overall impact. For example, healthy protein, fiber and good fats all influence the rate of sugar entry into the blood. Bottom line: if you're eating the Pyramid way, which is high in protein and fiber, no food—and that means watermelon and all other fruits—should be considered off-limits.

There's another consideration as well. As small incidental snacks, candies tend to be consumed almost mindlessly; they thus tempt us to eat more—more, certainly, than is shown in the demonstration. Eating more and more of these sugar-filled, nutrition-free items eventually mitigates against weight loss and diabetes prevention, while the fruit, with fiber, phytonutrients and a low calorie count, advances both those goals.

WHICH SNACK?

We've paired relatively small candy servings—and in one case a tart—with pretty good-sized servings of fruit. The calorie differences speak for themselves. That's true whether the fruit is raw, like the cherries, banana and cantaloupe, or cooked, as in the baked apple.

Bottom line? The sugar in fruit is great for satisfying your sweet craving without adding the calories that stymie weight loss and the fight against diabetes. In fact, the fiber and phytonutrients you'll take in with these fruit snacks will help you achieve both aims—weight loss and diabetes prevention or management.

And don't forget to check out the recipe for Tutti-Frutti Baked Apples (on page 120).

VS.

3 sticks red licorice
120 calories

1 cup cherries
50 calories

VS.

2 ounces gummy bears
200 calories

banana
100 calories

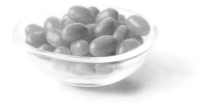

VS.

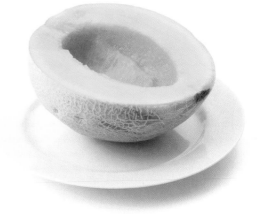

1½ ounces jelly beans
150 calories

½ cantaloupe
60 calories

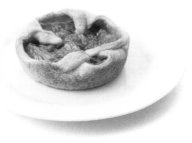

VS.

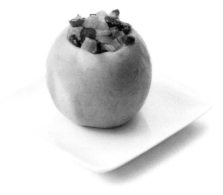

apple tart
390 calories

Tutti-Frutti Baked Apple
130 calories

SWEETS ON A STICK

No one is claiming that no-sugar-added frozen fudge pops, ice pops or fruit-and-cream pops contain any particular nutrients that will help you battle diabetes and lose weight. It's what these sweets *don't* contain that make them such important building blocks of the Beat Diabetes Pyramid: they don't have sugar, and they don't have fat.

And then, of course, they do contain one exceptionally important ingredient for any eating plan: their taste.

That makes these particular sweets extremely important in an overall eating plan aimed at weight loss and diabetes prevention or management: they satisfy that universal human sweet tooth without adding to either your waistline or your risk of this killer disease. **Bottom line?** *These no-added-sugar frozen treats can be enjoyed anytime, for any reason, in any quantity.*

Really? Really. Our nutritionist is adamant on this point. To those who object to buying these treats because they come in packages of a dozen and they're afraid they'll eat "more than one," she responds: "Feel free!" In fact, she says, even if you are diabetic, you can eat as many as you need to feel satisfied and still be ahead in the fight for weight loss and against diabetes. Those who indulge freely in these low-calorie treats tend to eat less of their high-calorie counterparts over time.

As you can see in the photograph, there is a very substantial range of these products. And if you still doubt that you can enjoy these products in an eating plan that advances weight loss and fights diabetes, check out the following food demonstrations.

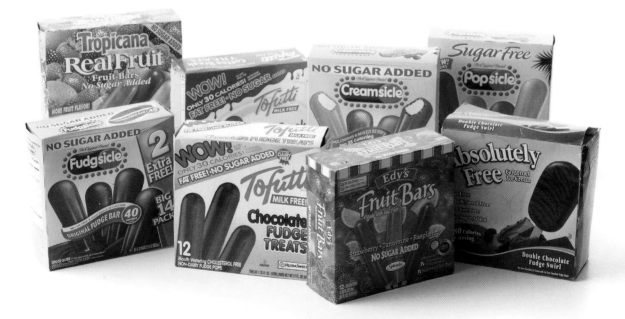

GENEROUS SERVING

Remember we said that the sweets on the top rung of the Beat Diabetes Pyramid should be eaten generously? Here's an example:

Between a bare mouthful of chocolate taste or one, two, three, even four Tofutti Chocolate Fudge Treats for the same calorie count, you can afford to be generous.

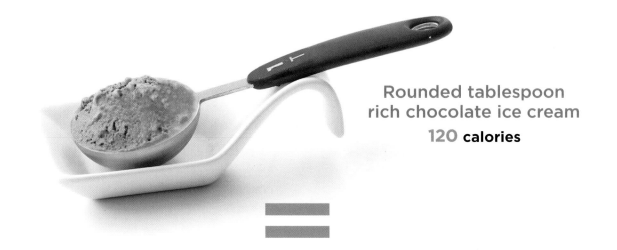

Rounded tablespoon
rich chocolate ice cream
120 calories

=

4 Tofutti Chocolate
Fudge Treats
120 calories

NO-ADDED-SUGAR CANDIES

There are times when you just need a quick hit of something sweet, and there is no dearth of no-added-sugar candies to meet that need—lollipops, gummy bears, sourballs, jelly beans, candy canes...you name it. For the most part, the candies on the Beat Diabetes Pyramid are hard candies or chewy fruit candies; these are lower in fat and calories than the nuggets or cream candies.

As with all the foods on the Pyramid, the watchword about how much to eat is "till satisfied." At least as far as weight loss and diabetes prevention are concerned, these candies are no exception. The sweeteners used in these candies are mostly sugar alcohols, which are both lower in calories than regular sugar and are much more slowly absorbed into the bloodstream. **Bottom line:** *they simply don't affect blood sugar levels in any appreciable way.*

There is one caveat about eating a lot of these candies, however, and it's often stated on the packaging: "excessive consumption may have a laxative effect." So if you're not used to eating these candies, go easy—at least at first.

OTHER SUGAR-FREE DESSERTS: ONE CAUTION

When buying—or baking—such other sugar-free desserts as cakes, pies, cookies, tarts and the like, there's one issue to keep in mind. *Although the food may lack sugar, it may well contain refined carbohydrates in the form of flour, and it might also have a fair amount of bad fat—neither of which helps you lose weight or prevent or control diabetes, as the picture about sugar-free cookies on page 183 makes clear.*

One reason is that *the human body processes flour and other starches much the same way it processes sugar.* After all, refined carbohydrate is refined carbohydrate—and the result for weight control and diabetes prevention is equivalent.

So it's important not to be taken in by the labeling; the "sugar-free" claim is true, but it doesn't tell the whole story. In fact, we sometimes refer to these foods as "saboteurs," because in the guise of doing good things for weight loss and your health, they actually subvert those goals.

Beware!

STRAWBERRY DRAMA

Check out the representations of fat and sugar content along with the calorie counts in these strawberry desserts. They tell a pretty dramatic story.

Note that to eat the calorie count of the scoop of ice cream, you would have to eat twenty-two of the frozen pops.

Be aware also that Italian ices and granitas are equivalent to the sorbet in this demonstration in terms of calories and sugar content.

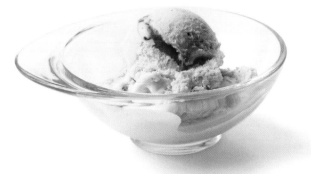
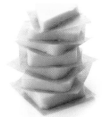
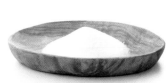

33 grams bad fat
= 6½ pats butter

12 teaspoons sugar

1-cup scoop rich strawberry ice cream
540 calories, **33** grams fat, **48** grams sugar

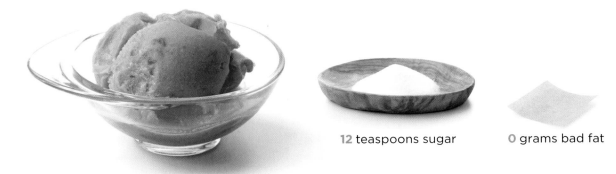

12 teaspoons sugar

0 grams bad fat

1-cup scoop strawberry sorbet
200 calories, **0** grams fat, **48** grams sugar

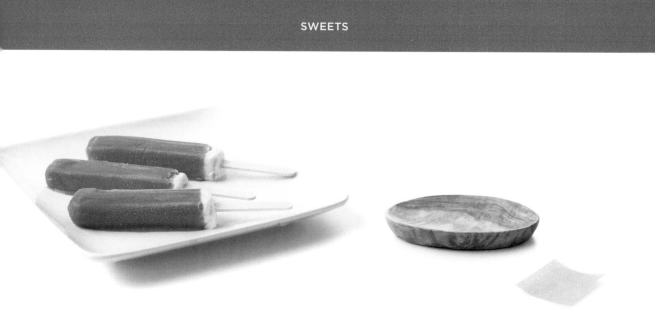

3 sugar-free strawberry Creamsicles
75 calories, 0 grams fat, 0 grams sugar

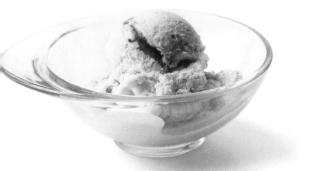

1-cup scoop rich
strawberry ice cream
540 calories

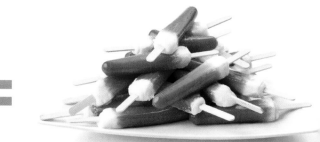

22 sugar-free strawberry
Creamsicles
**540 calories, 0 grams fat,
0 grams sugar**

LO-CAL SWEETENERS: NO FEAR!

If you have read horror stories about sweeteners in no-added-sugar treats, sugar-free candies or diet beverages, relax: the stories are not supported by scientific evidence. All sweeteners approved by the U.S. Food and Drug Administration (FDA) have been subjected to rigorous scrutiny, and we consider low-calorie sweeteners both safe and useful.

Useful they certainly are. Sweeteners are one area where "natural" is not necessarily better: sugars, honey and syrups are not helpful where both weight loss and fighting diabetes are concerned. So by all means, use the sweeteners to take the edge off a tart beverage, satisfy your sweet tooth or in cooking, and don't worry about them in the treats on the Beat Diabetes Pyramid.

For the most part, the dessert recipes in this book call for and have been tested with Splenda, but by all means follow your own lo-cal sweetener preference.

One caveat: we do not recommend aspartame—sold as NutraSweet or Equal—for use in *cooking,* although it's fine as an addition to a drink or sprinkled on your fruit.

A NOTE ON CHOCOLATE: THE GOOD KEEPS GETTING BETTER

Chocolate is the gift that keeps giving—as rich in health benefits as it is in pleasurable taste. Yes, chocolate contains saturated fat, but unlike other saturated fats, its fat content does not raise blood cholesterol levels. And cocoa, which is chocolate without the fat, is even low in calories.

We're talking here about dark chocolate—not milk or white chocolate, which are loaded with sugar. White chocolate, in fact, is not technically chocolate at all and delivers none of the considerable health benefits of chocolate.

But at the heart of the matter is chocolate's content of flavonols, phytonutrients found in many fruits and vegetables, including the cocoa bean. Especially where diabetes is an issue, flavonols pack a powerful health punch, helping to raise insulin sensitivity, lower blood pressure, decrease bad cholesterol, raise good cholesterol and promote the health of blood vessels. There's a simple way to put it: chocolate is very, very good for heart health.

Several studies have shown that insulin resistance drops and insulin sensitivity rises after ingesting chocolate—specifically, dark chocolate. That gives chocolate a special punch when it comes to preventing and/or managing diabetes.

Equally powerful is research showing chocolate's impact on blood pressure. One recent study demonstrated that the drop in blood pressure from consuming cocoa products was equivalent to the decrease that would have been achieved had the study participants been taking blood pressure medication! Well, how would you rather control your blood pressure—with prescription drugs or with cocoa?

Cocoa and chocolate have also been proven to be beneficial where vascular health is concerned. Studies have shown that these foods *help limit the buildup of plaque in the arteries by lowering LDL cholesterol. At the same time, they help raise HDL cholesterol levels.* Other studies demonstrate the power of chocolate to inhibit blood platelet activity and limit clotting—the same sort of thing aspirin does—and to keep the blood vessels relaxed and dilated, thus helping to maintain a healthy blood flow.

Yes, there are calories to contend with, so how can you get these stunning benefits of the flavonols without the calories? One answer is by focusing on cocoa—regular cocoa, not dutch cocoa, which is processed with an alkali that actually destroys the flavonols. Try adding a teaspoon of cocoa to your hot or iced coffee for a mocha effect. Or mix it into your sugar-free cocoa mix for a healthful hot chocolate on a cold winter's day. If you find the taste isn't sweet enough for you, add a packet or two of Splenda or your preferred low-calorie sweetener.

Another way to get the benefits of flavonols is sugar-free dark chocolate candy bars. Although caloric, these bars are fine for an occasional treat.

One note: when making desserts with chocolate, always use unsweetened or baking chocolate (100 percent cacao), and sweeten with sugar-free syrup, sugar-free preserves or the low-calorie sweetener of your choice.

As you see, chocolate can be your friend. And as the recipes that follow demonstrate, where weight loss and diabetes management are concerned, chocolate lovers really can have it all.

BEAT DIABETES BROWNIES

1 cup granulated Splenda

$\frac{1}{2}$ cup whole-wheat flour

$\frac{1}{2}$ cup unsweetened soy protein powder*

6-8 tablespoons unsweetened cocoa powder

$1\frac{1}{4}$ teaspoons baking powder

$\frac{1}{4}$ teaspoon salt

$\frac{2}{3}$ cup brewed coffee, regular or decaffeinated

$\frac{1}{2}$ cup sugar-free syrup (preferably chocolate, but any flavor is fine)

$\frac{1}{3}$ cup canola oil

1 tablespoon vanilla extract

$\frac{1}{2}$ cup coarsely chopped walnuts or pecans

Preheat oven to 350°F. Oil an 8- or 9-inch square baking pan, or coat with nonstick spray.

1. In a large bowl combine Splenda, flour, protein powder and salt. Add coffee, syrup, oil and vanilla, and stir until well blended.

2. Pour mixture into prepared pan. Sprinkle chopped nuts evenly over top and press gently into batter.

3. Bake 20–25 minutes, or until a toothpick inserted near the center comes out clean. Cool thoroughly in pan before cutting into squares.

Yield: 12 brownies

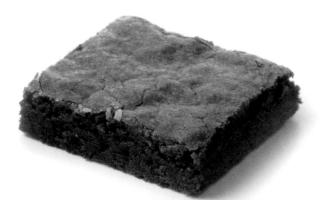

Regular brownie (2$\frac{1}{2}$ ounces)
360 calories, 14 grams fat, 20 grams sugar
= 3 pats butter, 5 teaspoons sugar

VS.

* Available in health-food stores and many markets (Whole Foods, Trader Joe's, etc.).

Beat Diabetes Brownie
(per 2½-ounce brownie)
110 calories
9 grams fiber
= no sugar added
less than 1 gram saturated fat

LEMON-BERRY PARFAIT

1 package sugar-free instant lemon pudding

1½ cups soy milk

2 tablespoons lemon juice

¼ teaspoon grated lemon zest

1½ cups sliced strawberries and/or raspberries

1. In a bowl, beat together pudding mix, soy milk and lemon juice, and zest until smooth.

2. Refrigerate for about 15 minutes to allow mixture to thicken slightly.

3. Divide pudding and berries evenly among 3 dessert dishes, alternating layers of pudding and berries.

Yield: 3 servings

105 calories per serving

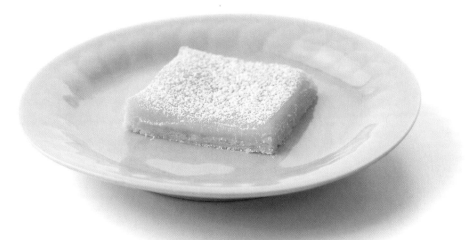

Lemon square (pastry)
420 calories, 0 grams fiber
20 grams fat = 4 pats butter
48 grams sugar = 12 teaspoons sugar

VS.

Lemon-Berry Parfait
105 calories
4 grams fiber
0 grams fat
0 grams sugar

BEAT DIABETES CHOCOLATE FONDUE

1 ounce unsweetened chocolate, chopped

1 ½ brewed cups coffee, regular or decaffeinated

1 cup soy milk

1 package sugar-free chocolate pudding mix, *not* instant

Pinch of salt

1 teaspoon vanilla extract

1 tablespoon rum or brandy, or 1 teaspoon flavoring (rum, almond, orange, maple, hazelnut, etc.)

1. Add chocolate and coffee to a medium saucepan. Stir mixture over low heat until chocolate is melted; remove from heat. Add soy milk, pudding mix and salt, and stir or whisk until mixture is smooth.

2. Cook over medium heat, stirring frequently, until mixture comes to a boil and begins to thicken. Stir in vanilla and rum or brandy, or other flavoring.

3. Serve warm, in a fondue pot, with assorted fruit.

Yield: about 6 ½-cup servings

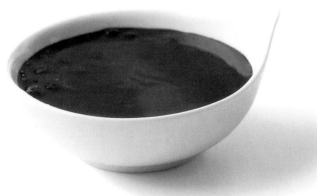

½ cup regular chocolate fondue
400 calories, 35 grams fat,
20 grams sugar
= 7 pats butter, 5 teaspoons sugar

VS.

*The saturated fat, represented by the butter, is from the chocolate in the recipe. The fat in chocolate, though it is saturated, does not raise blood cholesterol. The saturated fat in the regular fondue, however, is from both chocolate and cream; the latter does raise cholesterol.

118

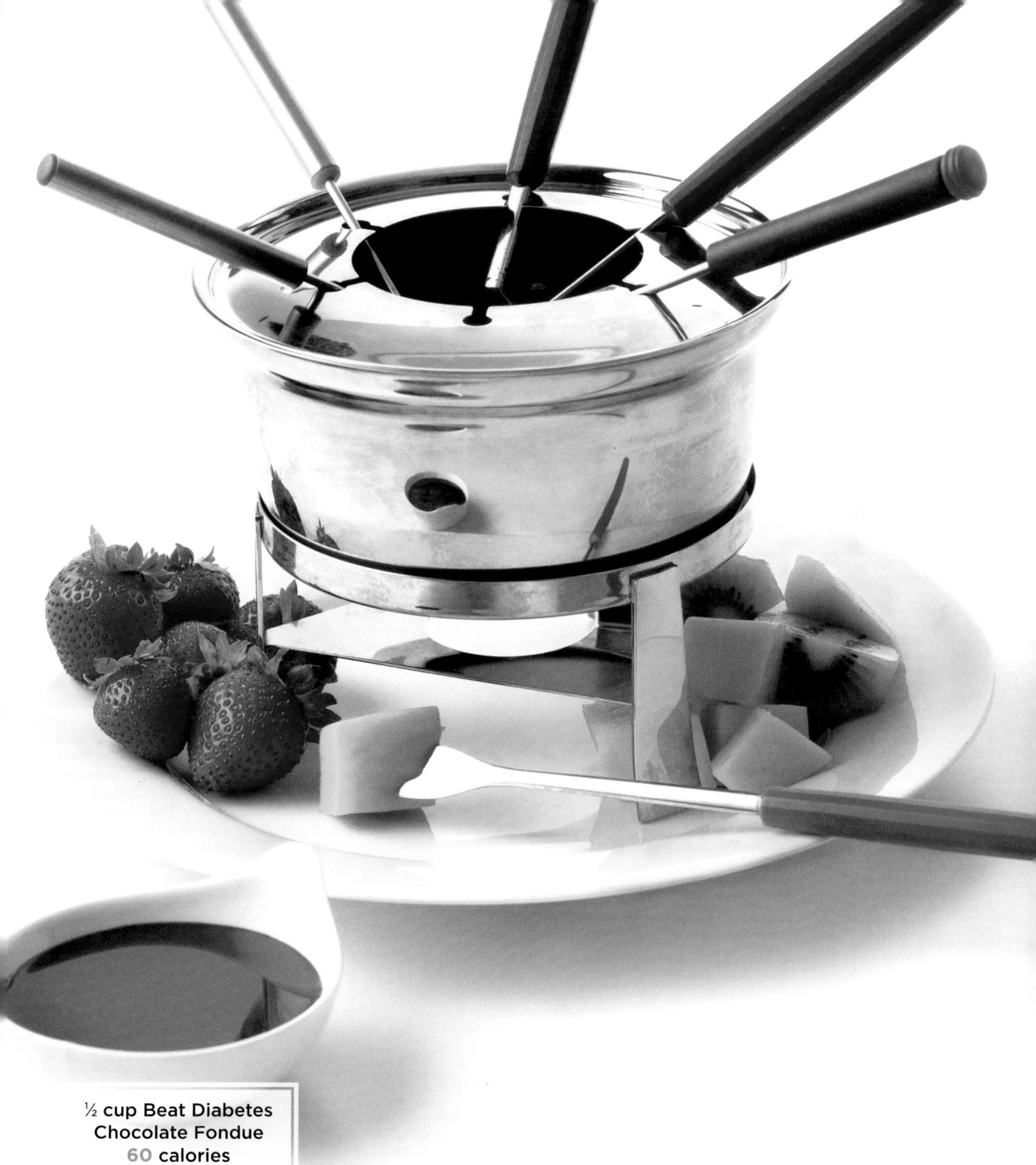

½ cup Beat Diabetes
Chocolate Fondue
60 calories
3 grams fat*
= ½ pat butter,
no sugar added

TUTTI-FRUTTI BAKED APPLE

4 large apples

1 cup diced mixed fruit, fresh or frozen (cherries, peaches, pineapple, etc.)

$\frac{1}{4}$ cup sugar-free jam or marmalade

2-3 packets Splenda

$\frac{1}{4}$ teaspoon cinnamon

Preheat oven to 350°F.

1. Core the apples and place in a 9-inch round or square baking pan.

2. Mix remaining ingredients together in a bowl.

3. Fill the apples with the fruit mixture, mounding any additional fruit on top of each apple.

4. Add a few tablespoons of water to the pan and cover with foil.

5. Bake 30 minutes; remove the foil and bake an additional 15 minutes, or until apples are tender. Serve warm or cold.

Yield: 4 servings

130 calories each

VS.

Apple tart
390 calories

Tutti-Frutti Baked Apple
130 calories

120

CHAPTER 9

Look and Lose

See for yourself.

Everything we've been telling you in the past eight chapters—all the science and all the background detail on the various kinds of food—goes into action in the pages that follow. Here you'll find the kind of Picture Perfect demonstrations that have long been the signature trademark of Dr. Shapiro's bestselling books.

What are Picture Perfect demonstrations? They're vivid comparisons of related food options and the health and weight-management consequences of each option. One look and you get the picture—perfectly. And once that picture is in your brain, you never forget it.

Some of it will surprise you. Maybe for years you've been depriving yourself of pancakes slathered in syrup—way too fattening, you assumed. Have a look at the Monarch's Meal demo and think again. Or maybe you've been careful to satisfy your coffee craving with a no-fat, no-cream version that still gratifies your sweet tooth. Is it Place Your Order? Check out the demo by that name to see the truth.

In the gallery of demonstrations that follow, you'll see the truth for yourself in comparisons of breakfasts, lunches, snacks, appetizers, dinners, desserts and saboteur foods. No one is telling you what to eat. But it's been proven time and again that once you see what each option really represents—and what the consequences can be to your waistline and your health—you'll know which choice is right for you.

BIG IS BEAUTIFUL

You'll pay a big price in calories and heart health for this small breakfast of a muffin and chai. Filled with sugar and fat, it's a diabetes grenade waiting for the pin to be pulled. The exact opposite is true for the breakfast on the right—waffles smothered in sugar-free syrup, plus blueberries, plus coffee laced with milk. With a fraction of the calories, fat and sugar of the small breakfast, and with more than ten times as much fiber, this big breakfast is definitely beautiful.

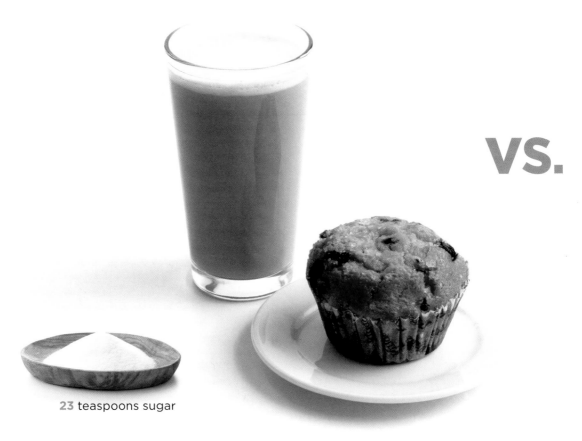

VS.

23 teaspoons sugar

5-ounce blueberry muffin	550 **calories**	10 **grams fat**	1 **gram fiber**	52 **grams sugar**
Medium chai latte	290 **calories**	7 **grams fat**	0 **grams fiber**	39 **grams sugar**
TOTAL	840 calories	17 grams fat	1 gram fiber	91 grams sugar

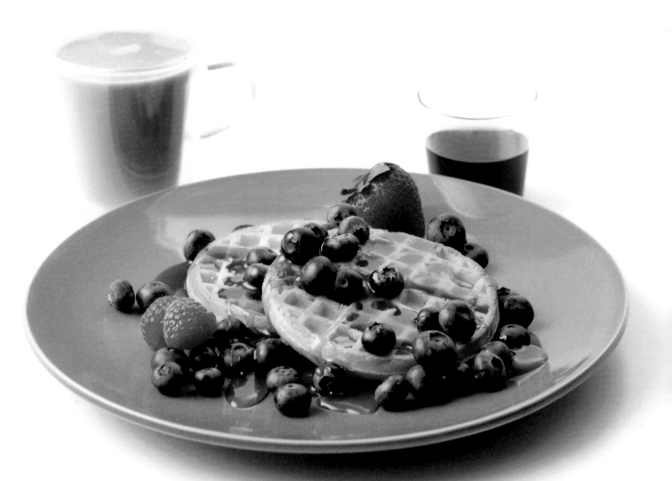

2 Van's waffles	150 calories	3½ grams fat	8 grams fiber	3 grams sugar
2 tablespoons sugar-free syrup	10 calories	0 grams fat	0 grams fiber	0 grams sugar
⅓ cup blueberries	25 calories	0 grams fat	3 grams fiber	0 grams sugar
Coffee with low-cal sweetener, 2 tablespoons milk	20 calories	0 grams fat	0 grams fiber	0 grams sugar

TOTAL **205** calories **3½** grams fat **11** grams fiber **3** grams sugar

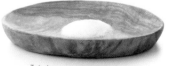

¾ teaspoon sugar

SWEET TOOTH AT BREAKFAST

If you're someone who likes to start the day with a sweet taste in your mouth, you don't have to do it at peril to your waistline and your health. Check out the calorie difference between the single cranberry scone and four—count 'em!—pieces of light bread slathered with sugar-free jam. Get your fiber, avoid the fat and satisfy your sweet tooth four times over with this choice of breakfast.

5-ounce cranberry scone	**500 calories**	**20 grams fat**	**0 grams fiber**
1-ounce butter (2 tablespoons)	**220 calories**	**25 grams fat**	**0 grams fiber**
TOTAL	**720** calories	**45** grams fat	**0** grams fiber

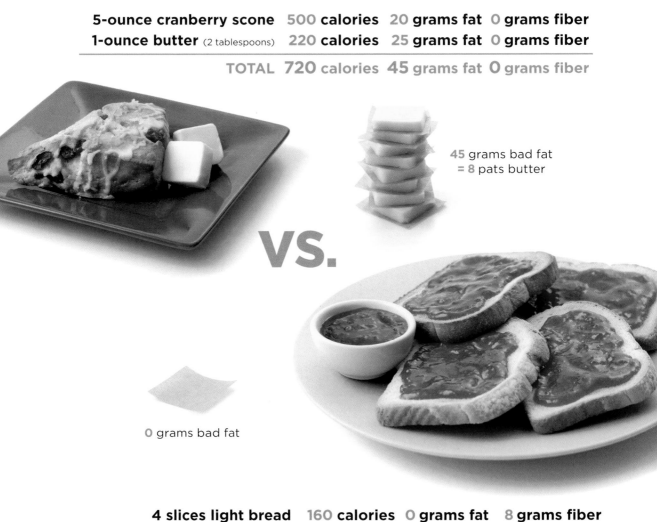

45 grams bad fat
= 8 pats butter

VS.

0 grams bad fat

4 slices light bread	**160 calories**	**0 grams fat**	**8 grams fiber**
4 tablespoons sugar-free jam	**40 calories**	**0 grams fat**	**0 grams fiber**
TOTAL	**200** calories	**0** grams fat	**8** grams fiber

SABOTAGE IN THE MORNING

Ah, granola! So natural! So filled with fiber! So good for you! Well...look again.

Granola is a classic saboteur food. For the 8 grams of fiber this natural breakfast food provides, you pay a high price in the sugar and calories that can add weight and play havoc with your blood sugar levels. How about tripling the fiber content of your breakfast with no sugar at all? That's what the cereal breakfast below provides.

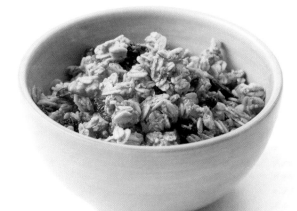

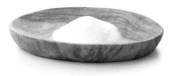

1 cup granola
520 calories, **8** grams fiber, **28** grams sugar

VS.

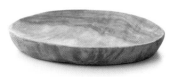

1 cup All-Bran Extra Fiber or Fiber One
100 calories, **28** grams fiber, **0** grams sugar

KEEPING UP TRADITION

The sausage biscuit is an all-American tradition. But it's a tradition that comes with enough saturated fat and refined carbohydrates to kick metabolic syndrome into high gear. So is there a diabetes-fighting way to get the traditional taste? You're looking at it below.

4-ounce biscuit	400	**calories**	20	**grams fat**	0	**grams fiber**
1 40-gram sausage patty	135	**calories**	12	**grams fat**	0	**grams fiber**
TOTAL	535	calories	32	grams fat	0	grams fiber

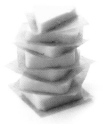

32 grams bad fat
= 6 ½ pats butter

VS.

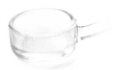

3 grams good fat
= ½ teaspoon oil

Light English muffin	100	**calories**	0	**grams fat**	6	**grams fiber**
1 40-gram veggie sausage patty	80	**calories**	3	**grams fat**	3	**grams fiber**
TOTAL	180	calories	3	grams fat	9	grams fiber

CONVENIENCE FACTOR

There it is: the lone buttered bagel, the quick and easy breakfast for folks on the move. But in this particular case, convenience costs you—in a ridiculously high number of calories and fat grams. Just as convenient would be a slice of light wheat toast with peanut butter. It contains one-fourth of the bagel's calories and fat. Plus, it's full of diabetes- and weight-fighting fiber. And it would take a tower of these bread slices to equal that poor lone bagel.

5-ounce bagel	400 **calories**	0 **grams fat**
2 tablespoons butter	220 **calories**	24 **grams fat**
TOTAL	620 calories	24 grams fat

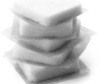

24 grams bad fat
= 5 pats butter

16 grams good fat
= 3 teaspoons oil

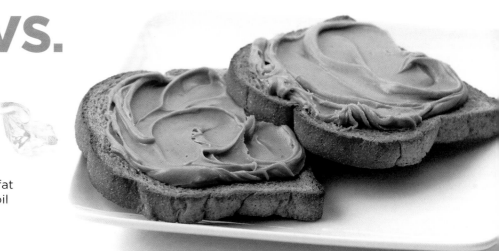

2 slices light wheat toast	80 **calories**	0 **grams fat**
2 tablespoons peanut butter	190 **calories**	16 **grams fat**
TOTAL	270 calories	16 grams fat

MONARCH'S MEAL

Take a quick look at these two breakfasts—the bagel with cream cheese and the regal meal of pancakes with syrup, sausage *and* melon—and you'd probably figure that the better choice for weight loss and health would be the bagel. But you'd be wrong. For starters, look at the calorie difference. But don't stop there. While calories and fat are all the bagel offers—too much of both—the royal feast is filled with diabetes fighters such as fiber and even soy protein. So do as royalty does and choose this breakfast fit for a king.

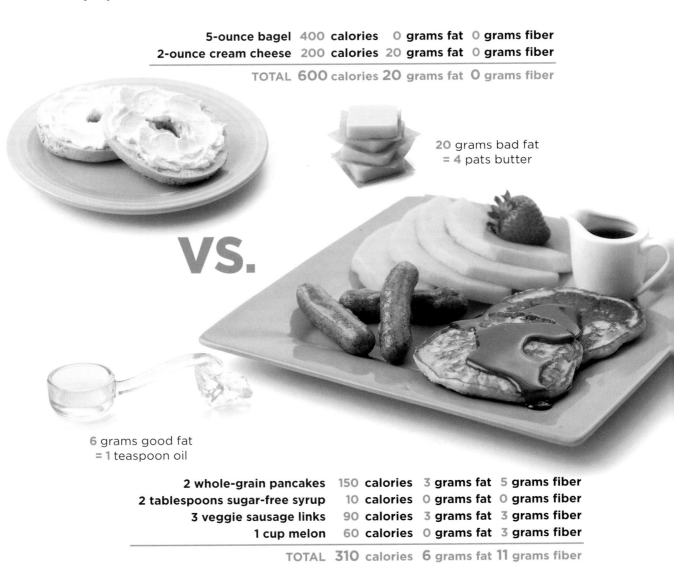

5-ounce bagel	400 **calories**	0 **grams fat**	0 **grams fiber**
2-ounce cream cheese	200 **calories**	20 **grams fat**	0 **grams fiber**
TOTAL	600 calories	20 grams fat	0 grams fiber

20 grams bad fat
= 4 pats butter

6 grams good fat
= 1 teaspoon oil

2 whole-grain pancakes	150 **calories**	3 **grams fat**	5 **grams fiber**
2 tablespoons sugar-free syrup	10 **calories**	0 **grams fat**	0 **grams fiber**
3 veggie sausage links	90 **calories**	3 **grams fat**	3 **grams fiber**
1 cup melon	60 **calories**	0 **grams fat**	3 **grams fiber**
TOTAL	310 calories	6 grams fat	11 grams fiber

VARIATIONS ON A CLASSIC

The sandwich is perhaps the classic lunch—its variations limited only by the imagination. It's also a perfect opportunity for the imagination to choose variations that can help you lose weight and prevent, fight or manage diabetes. Take a look.

Get a load of the off-the-charts calorie count on this ham and cheese on a croissant and the simple egg salad on a bagel on the next page. Moreover, these calories come mostly in the form of refined carbohydrates, saturated fat and cholesterol—bad choices if you're health-conscious, and especially if you want to manage your weight and fight diabetes.

With roast beef on a roll and turkey on rye, you can manage to lower the calorie count because these sandwiches are somewhat lower in saturated fat and carbohydrates. But not that much—certainly not enough for weight management and fighting diabetes.

We've slashed the calorie count with these two sandwiches—tuna salad (made with light mayo) on whole-wheat bread and veggie deli on light bread, both with lettuce and tomato, both delicious. But that's not all. Both of these sandwiches are also made with ingredients found on the Beat Diabetes Pyramid and offer virtually no saturated fat and lots of fiber. The tuna salad gives you omega-3 fatty acids with your protein, while the veggie deli sandwich provides the extra added attraction of soy protein, which is just about the most powerful weapon you can find for heart health and against diabetes.

For your weight and your health, these two Pyramid sandwiches are as good as it gets. They deserve the name "classics."

6 sandwiches—worst to best

Ham and cheese on a croissant

3½-ounce croissant	390 **calories**
3 ounces ham	195 **calories**
3 ounces American cheese	300 **calories**
TOTAL	885 calories

Egg salad on a bagel

4-ounce bagel 320 **calories**
1 cup egg salad 440 **calories**

TOTAL **760** calories

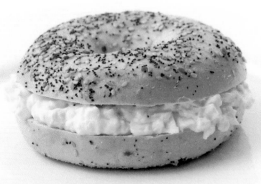

Roast beef on a roll

2½-ounce kaiser roll 200 **calories**
6 ounces roast beef 390 **calories**
1 tablespoon catsup 15 **calories**

TOTAL **605** calories

Turkey on rye

2 slices rye bread	160 **calories**
6 ounces white-meat turkey	300 **calories**
1 tablespoon mayo	100 **calories**
TOTAL 560 calories	

Light tuna salad on whole wheat
with lettuce and tomato

2 slices whole-wheat bread	140 **calories**
6 ounces tuna salad made with light mayo	250 **calories**
Lettuce and tomato	5 **calories**
TOTAL 395 calories	

131

Veggie deli on light bread
with lettuce and tomato

2 slices light wheat bread	**80 calories**
6 ounces veggie deli	**180 calories**
Lettuce and tomato	**5 calories**
1 tablespoon mustard	**10 calories**

TOTAL 275 calories

BARGAIN SHOPPING

With their endless possibilities for adding yet one more ingredient or condiment, soups are a real bargain—a great way to fill up deliciously on lots of healthy foods that are good sources of fiber and phytonutrients. But here, too, the choices you make are significant. Check out the four soups on the next page. All fill you with calories—mostly from refined carbohydrates and/ or saturated fat—and all provide less than a single gram of fiber per serving. The soups on the bottom, however, are all Pyramid soups; they contain legumes and vegetables straight from the Beat Diabetes Pyramid, are low in refined carbohydrates and saturated fat, are virtually cholesterol-free and provide anywhere from 6 to 9 grams of fiber per serving.

Bottom line: if you're going for a bargain, shop carefully.

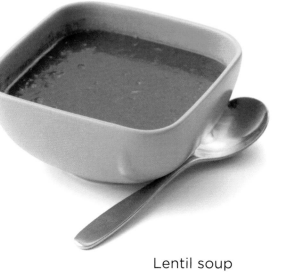

New England clam chowder   Ramen noodle soup
Cream of mushroom soup   French onion soup
Seafood bisque   Chicken rice soup

Calories from refined carbs and/or saturated fat
Less than 1 gram of fiber per serving

Lentil soup   Carrot-ginger soup
Split pea soup   Black bean soup
Tomato vegetable soup   Manhattan clam chowder

Low in refined carbs and saturated fat
6-9 grams fiber per serving

TUNA TODAY

It's the great lunch standby: a tuna salad sandwich. But if you choose wisely, you can turn the standby into the gold standard of diabetes-fighting lunches. Tuna salad on a baguette? High in calories, 1 gram of fiber, not that filling a lunch. Light-mayo tuna salad on whole wheat with sliced tomato? Just about half the calories, *plus* 10 grams of fiber, *plus* phytonutrients—a triple punch against weight gain and diabetes. Add a bowl of chunky vegetable soup for more fiber, and you still won't come close to the calorie hit of the tuna on a baguette.

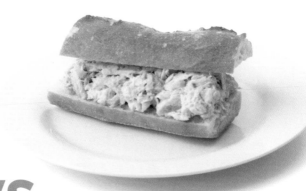

Tuna on a baguette

¾ cup tuna salad	**330 calories**
5-ounce baguette	**400 calories**
TOTAL	**730** calories

VS.

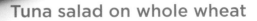

Tuna salad on whole wheat

¾ cup tuna salad (with light mayo)	**225 calories**
2 slices whole-wheat bread	**140 calories**
2 slices tomato	**5 calories**
Bowl of chunky vegetable soup	**100 calories**
TOTAL	**470** calories

HOT DOG!

Grab a quick hot dog and what do you get? Calories and fat—and you're still hungry. Here's an alternative.

A veggie frank on a light bun has the same taste and same condiments—at a third of the calories, no fat, with 3 grams of fiber. Still hungry? How about a baked potato with bean chili? Your total calorie count now equals the one quick hot dog, but you're losing the fat and gaining plenty of fiber.

Frankfurter	180 **calories**	17 **grams fat**	0 **grams fiber**
Bun	120 **calories**	0 **grams fat**	0 **grams fiber**
Mustard and relish	10 **calories**	0 **grams fat**	0 **grams fiber**
TOTAL	**310** calories	**2** grams fat	**0** grams fiber

=

Veggie frank	40 **calories**	0 **grams fat**	1 **gram fiber**
Light bun	80 **calories**	0 **grams fat**	2 **grams fiber**
Mustard and relish	10 **calories**	0 **grams fat**	0 **grams fiber**
Baked potato	120 **calories**	0 **grams fat**	2½ **grams fiber**
¼ cup bean chili	60 **calories**	1 **gram fat**	3 **grams fiber**
TOTAL	**310** calories	**1** gram fat	**8½** grams fiber

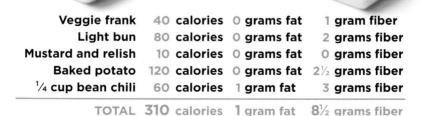

SALAD FOR LUNCH

Eleven and a half pats of butter: that's what you'll be burdening your waistline and your heart with when this small portion of chicken salad and Muenster cheese is your lunch. The 58 grams of fat in this calorie-heavy meal are mainly saturated fat, the kind that can raise your total and LDL cholesterol levels and burden your insulin receptors, thus raising the risk of diabetes.

Here's another salad—bigger than the high-fat one, more colorful, much more healthful and wonderfully tasty. Rich in protein from the seafood and in phytonutrients from the vegetables, it brings you the diabetes-fighting benefits of fiber at a low, low calorie count. And compare its single teaspoon of unsaturated fat with those eleven and a half pats of butter!

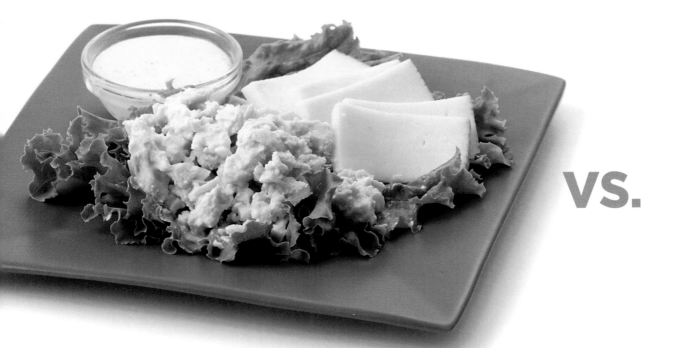

VS.

¾ cup chicken salad	360 calories	24 grams fat	½ gram fiber
2 ounces Muenster cheese	210 calories	17 grams fat	0 grams fiber
Lettuce	5 calories	0 grams fat	½ gram fiber
2 tablespoons ranch dressing	160 calories	17 grams fat	0 grams fiber
TOTAL	735 calories	58 grams fat	1 gram fiber

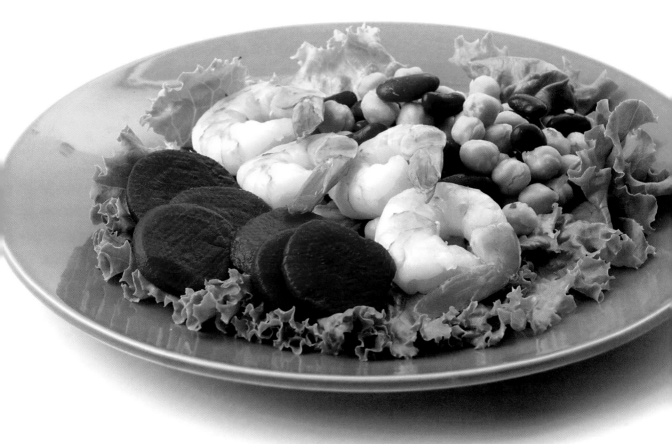

¾ cup bean salad	170 calories	3 grams fat	10 grams fiber
2 ounces seafood	60 calories	1 gram fat	0 grams fiber
⅓ cup sliced beets	10 calories	0 grams fat	1½ grams fiber
Lettuce	5 calories	0 grams fat	½ gram fiber
2 tablespoons light creamy dressing	20 calories	2 grams fat	0 grams fiber
TOTAL	**265** calories	**6** grams fat	**12** grams fiber

BEATING CAESAR

Edamame, the fresh green soybean, is among the hottest of the trendy new "designer foods," yet it has been cultivated across Asia as both food and medicine for some five thousand years. The current vogue for edamame seems to have been launched in Japan, where it gained popularity as a bar snack, typically served boiled and salted. Today, it's available in American supermarkets and gourmet shops in both fresh and frozen versions, and its pungent taste and crisp texture have made edamame a welcome ingredient in a range of dishes. This colorful recipe features edamame but blends a variety of tastes and textures, and it's a nutritionist's dream as well. The soy is an excellent source of protein, fiber and disease-fighting phytochemicals; the other vegetables—bell pepper, cucumber, scallion—add more nutrients; and the dressing, featuring both canola and sesame oil, offers just 7 grams of the best kind of fat. Caesar salad made with 3 ounces of chicken seems old hat by comparison, while its calorie count and fat content show it is not as benign as it looks.

EDAMAME SALAD

1 pound edamame (frozen blanched shelled soybeans)

3 tablespoons seasoned rice wine vinegar

2 tablespoons light soy sauce

1 teaspoon canola oil

1 teaspoon sesame oil

¼ teaspoon red pepper flakes

4 scallions, sliced diagonally

1 medium cucumber, peeled, halved, seeded and chopped

1 medium red bell pepper, chopped

Lettuce leaves

1. In a large pot over high heat, bring 6 cups salted water to a boil. Add the edamame and cook for 5 minutes, or until tender. Drain well.

2. Meanwhile, in a large bowl, whisk together the vinegar, soy sauce, canola oil, sesame oil and red pepper flakes. Add the drained soybeans, scallions, cucumber and bell pepper. Toss to coat. Serve on a bed of lettuce.

Yield: 6 servings

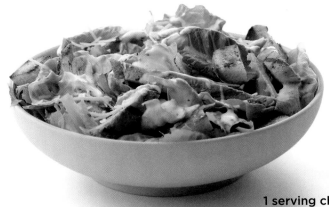

1 serving chicken
Caesar salad
450 calories
24 grams fat

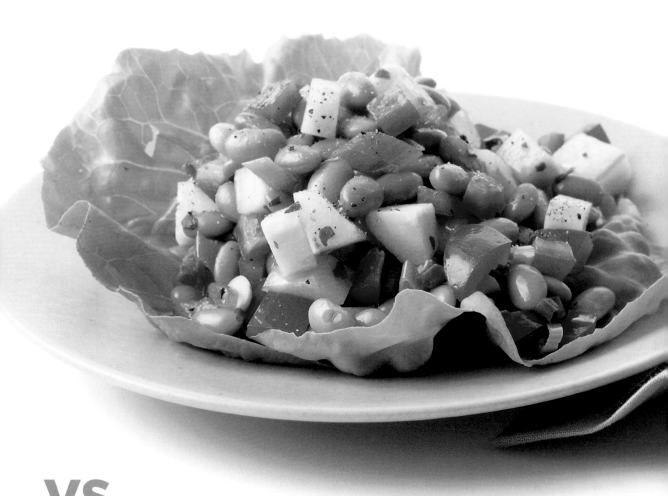

VS.

1 serving
Edamame Salad
106 calories
7 grams fat

SLOPPY BUT SLENDER

You can't see a difference between these two sloppy joes. Can't taste a difference, either. But if you're weight-conscious and health-conscious, you can measure the difference. The one on the left, made with veggie crumbles and on a light bun, has about half the calories of the one on the right and one-fifth of the fat. It also provides nine times the fiber content of the one on the right. Both joes may be sloppy, but the one on the left is managing his weight and fighting diabetes at the same time.

Bun	110 **calories**	0 **grams fat**	0 **grams fiber**
Sloppy joe mix with 6 ounces ground beef	480 **calories**	36 **grams fat**	0 **grams fiber**
½ **cup sauce**	70 **calories**	0 **grams fat**	1 **gram fiber**
TOTAL	**660** calories	**36** grams fat	**1** gram fiber

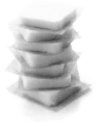

36 grams bad fat
= 7 pats butter

VS.

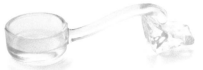

7 grams good fat
= 1½ teaspoons oil

Light bun	80 **calories**	0 **grams fat**	2 **grams fiber**
Sloppy joe mix with 6 ounces veggie crumbles	240 **calories**	7 **grams fat**	6 **grams fiber**
½ **cup sauce**	70 **calories**	0 **grams fat**	1 **gram fiber**
TOTAL	**390** calories	**7** grams fat	**9** grams fiber

MINDLESS SNACKS

They're the kinds of foods we tend to eat mindlessly. We just grab a handful of whatever snack is there—virtually without thinking. But with a little thought we can help maintain a healthy weight and fight diabetes at the same time. Take a look: one mindless snack, the tiny piece of cheese, is loaded with the kind of saturated fat that raises your risk of diabetes. But if you grab a handful of pistachios instead, you'll be taking in monounsaturated fat, which can actually help you prevent diabetes. So it doesn't take a lot of thought to get and stay healthy and diabetes-free.

3 ounces brie
342 calories, 27 grams fat

27 grams bad fat
= 5 ½ pats butter

2 ounces pistachios in shell
324 calories, 27 grams fat

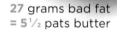

27 grams good fat
= 5 ½ teaspoons oil

WHICH WEDGE?

Even with two crackers, this slender wedge of white cheddar doesn't offer as much to eat as a single wedge of the pizza. And since it brings with it a huge calorie count, a high content of saturated fats and the dubious health effects of a dairy food, consider the pizza instead. You could have four wedges for the same cost in calories—and enjoy a range of tastes into the bargain.

CARAMELIZED ONION AND ROASTED RED PEPPER PIZZA

1 tablespoon olive oil

2 large onions, halved and thinly sliced

½ teaspoon salt

1 12-ounce jar roasted red peppers, drained, patted dry and coarsely chopped

2 tablespoons balsamic vinegar

5 whole-wheat pitas or flatbreads (8 inches each)

⅓ cup (1½ ounces) freshly shaved Parmesan cheese or dairy-free alternative

¼ cup loosely packed fresh basil leaves, cut into strips

Preheat the oven to 400°F.

1. Heat the oil in a large nonstick skillet over medium heat. Add the onions and salt and cook, stirring occasionally, for 20 minutes, or until very tender and golden brown. Stir in the peppers and vinegar.

2. Place the pitas or flatbreads on a baking sheet. Evenly divide the onion mixture among the pitas and sprinkle with the cheese. Bake for 10 minutes, or until the pitas are crisp. Remove the pizzas from the oven and sprinkle with the basil. To serve, cut each pizza into quarters.

Yield: 20 wedges

Per wedge: 80 calories, 2 grams fat

1 wedge (3 ounces)
white cheddar cheese
320 calories 28 grams fat

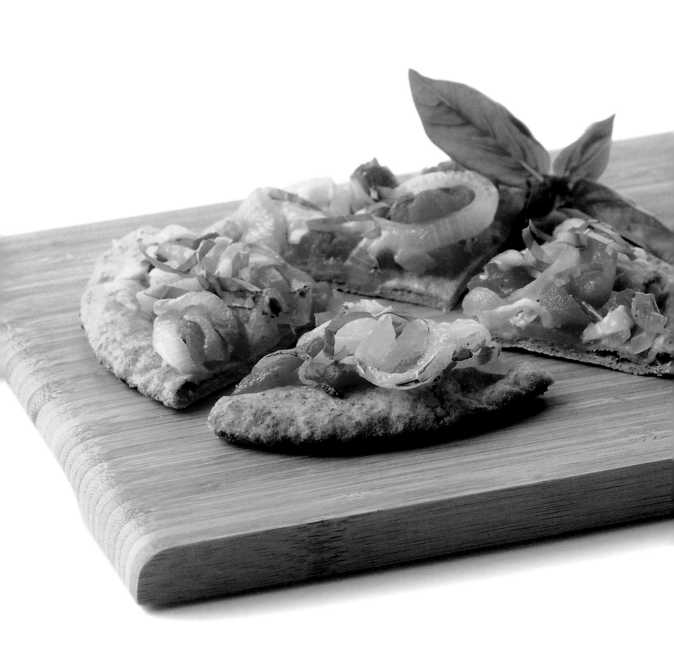

4 servings
Caramelized Onion and
Roasted Red Pepper Pizza
320 calories 8 grams fat

PEPPERONI PROMISE

Like pepperoni? Even a modest portion of small slices can be a high-calorie, high-fat snack. Or you can enjoy the taste you crave the low-calorie, no-fat way with veggie pepperoni that also offers you the diabetes-fighting benefits of soy protein. Add in some protein-filled shrimp, and you're still nowhere near the calorie cost of the meat pepperoni on its own.

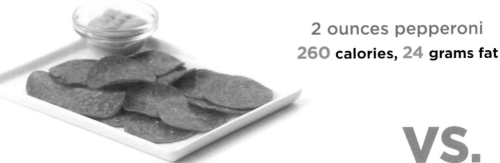

2 ounces pepperoni
260 calories, **24** grams fat

VS.

and

2 ounces veggie pepperoni	**80** calories	**0** grams fat
2 ounces shrimp	**60** calories	**1** gram fat
TOTAL	**140** calories	**1** gram fat

THE DISH ON DIPS

This may look like a choice between different kinds of dips, but it's also a choice between different kinds of fat. On the top are two dips with the kind of fat that can raise your cholesterol and your risk of diabetes—trans fat in the ranch dip and saturated fat in the blue cheese dip. On the bottom are two dips that can actually help prevent diabetes; both the hummus and the guacamole contain monounsaturated fat, one of the good fats. But that's not all. The ingredients in all the dips on the bottom are from the Beat Diabetes Pyramid—chickpeas and sesame tahini in the hummus and avocado in the guacamole—so you're actually fighting diabetes when you dip into them.

23 grams bad fat
= 4 ½ pats butter

Blue cheese dip (2 tablespoons)	160 **calories**	14 **grams fat**
Ranch dip (2 tablespoons)	172 **calories**	9 **grams fat**
	TOTAL	332 calories	23 grams fat

VS.

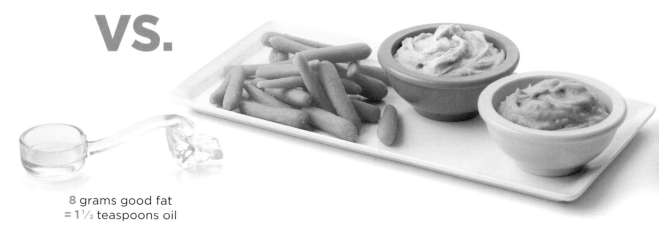

8 grams good fat
= 1 ½ teaspoons oil

Hummus (2 tablespoons)	52 **calories**	3 **grams fat**
Guacamole (2 tablespoons)	55 **calories**	5 **grams fat**
	TOTAL	107 calories	8 grams fat

IT'S YOUR PARTY!

Party mixes are hard to resist. Fail to resist the Chex Mix on the left, and you're taking in 242 calories and nearly 10 grams of fat. Yield to the soy crisps on the right, however, and you minimize your calorie and fat cost *and* give yourself the diabetes-fighting power of soy protein.

1⅓ **cups Chex Mix**
(2 ounces)

242 calories, 10 grams fat

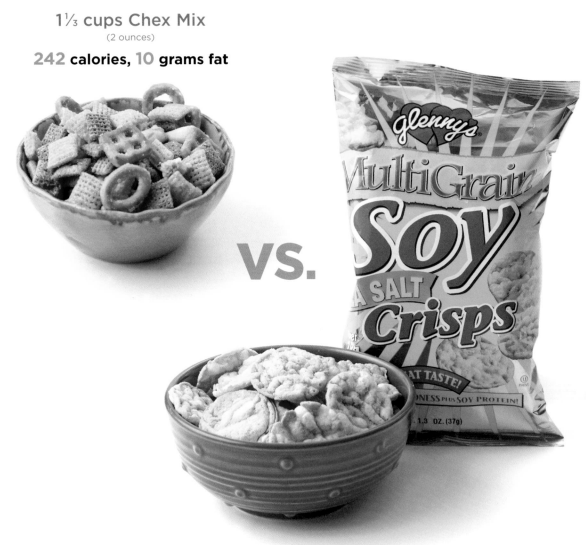

VS.

1.3-ounce bag Glenny's Soy Crisps
140 calories, 3 grams fat, 9 grams soy protein

EASY FIX

Crackers and cheese are an easy snack to prepare but very tough on your waistline and your health. Just check out the cost in fat grams and calories—mostly from refined carbohydrates—of these half dozen crackers with Swiss. The peanuts and olives snack is even easier to prepare, costs you about half the calories, contains healthy monounsaturated fat and adds the proactive power of fiber to your fight for weight loss and against diabetes.

6 Ritz crackers	105 **calories**	6 **grams fat**	0 **grams fiber**
3 ounces Swiss cheese	320 **calories**	24 **grams fat**	0 **grams fiber**
TOTAL	425 calories	30 grams fat	0 grams fiber

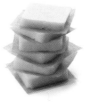

30 grams bad fat
= 6 pats butter

VS.

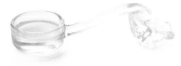

4 grams good fat
= 4 teaspoons oil

1-ounce peanuts in shell	160 **calories**	14 **grams fat**	2 **grams fiber**
15 large olives	70 **calories**	7 **grams fat**	2 **grams fiber**
TOTAL	230 calories	21 grams fat	4 grams fiber

EAT YOUR CALORIES, DON'T DRINK THEM

That's always a good idea: get your calories in filling foods rather than in beverages that are an accompaniment to additional meal items. And as this demonstration dramatically shows, it would take four oranges to equal the calorie count of this one glass of orange juice. So clearly, you're better off getting your orange taste by eating an orange rather than drinking its juice. But if you want your fruit taste in liquid form, try a tall, cool glass of a fruit-taste diet beverage—or any other diet beverage, for that matter.

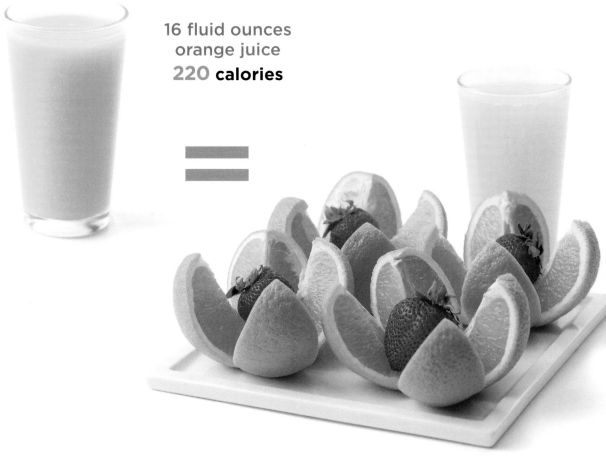

**16 fluid ounces
orange juice
220 calories**

16 fluid ounces Crystal Light   **5 calories**
4 oranges   **215 calories**
TOTAL 220 calories

PLACE YOUR ORDER

Even that nonfat venti-sized iced vanilla latte will cost you 240 calories, mostly in milk and sugar. Here's a weight-loss and diabetes-fighting tip: instead order a venti iced coffee with sugar-free vanilla syrup, then add a small amount of milk. Total calorie count? A mere 20 calories—for the same taste sensation.

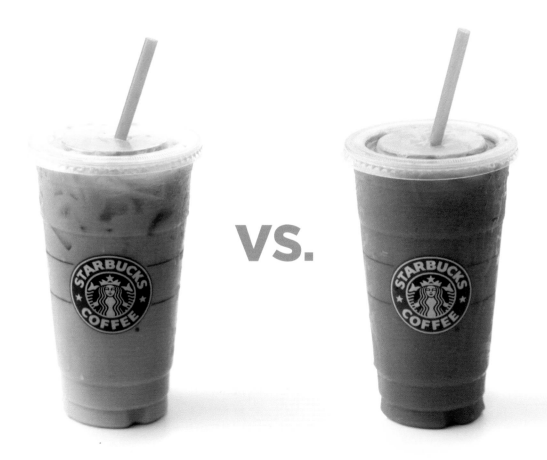

Nonfat venti iced vanilla latte
240 calories

VS.

Venti iced coffee with sugar-free vanilla syrup and 2 tablespoons whole milk
20 calories

SHAKE IT UP!

Get your healthy, natural yogurt or whey protein shake here! Naturally sweetened with natural honey! Well, all that natural so-called goodness will cost you 350 calories and a truckload of sugar. And the dairy you take in is no friend to your efforts to fight diabetes. Instead, make your shake with a soy protein powder, sweeten it with a low-calorie sweetener, and know that you have saved yourself 200 calories and are battling diabetes with soy, just about the strongest weapon there is against this killer disease.

Yogurt or whey protein shake sweetened with honey
350 calories, 69 grams sugar

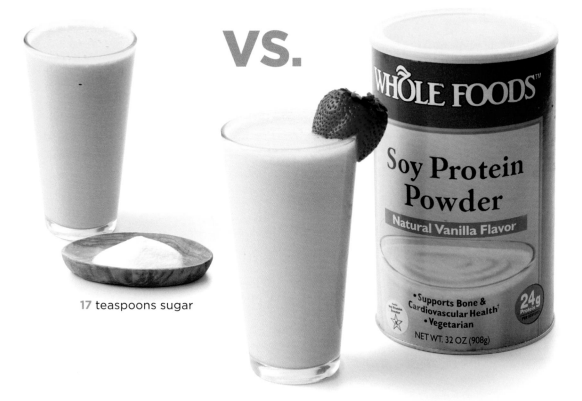

VS.

17 teaspoons sugar

Soy protein shake with Splenda and ½ cup of strawberries
150 calories, 0 grams sugar

SIZE MATTERS

These three mini quiches stuffed with ham and cheese barely take the edge off your appetite. Yet for the same number of calories, you can enjoy this feast of crabmeat-filled tomatoes. The striking difference in the amount of food becomes even more striking when you see how much you're saving in fat intake—and how much fiber and phytonutrients you're gaining with the tomato-and-crabmeat appetizers.

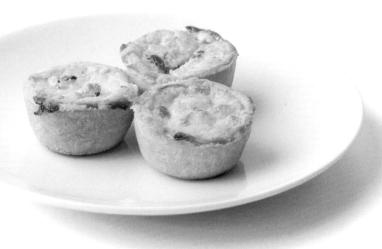

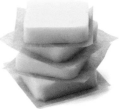

20 grams bad fat
= **4** pats butter

3 ham-and-cheese mini quiches (3 ounces)
215 calories, 20 grams fat

=

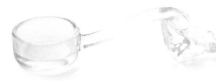

2 grams good fat
= ¹⁄₂ teaspoon oil

10 plum tomatoes filled with 6 ounces crabmeat
215 calories, 2 grams fat

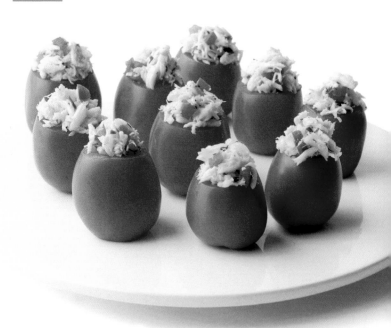

CREAMY GOLDEN SOUP

When what you crave is a creamy, golden-yellow soup, go for the one with the nutrition benefits and the calorie savings. This curried yellow split pea soup hits the spot when you're in the mood for something smooth and rich, and it brings you the rewards of phytonutrients as well— without the high calorie count and saturated fat content of the cheese soup.

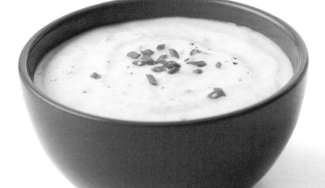

45 grams bad fat
= 9 pats butter

1 cup 4-cheese soup
470 calories, 45 grams fat

VS.

2 grams good fat
= ½ teaspoon oil

**1 cup curried yellow
split pea soup**
150 calories, 2 grams fat, 4 grams fiber

A CROWDED PLATTER OF TASTE AND NUTRITION

Those lonely-looking cubes of cheese and pâté contain a whopping 375 calories and represent a pile of fat. Check out instead the crowded platter of elegant smoked salmon with cucumbers— at far fewer calories and less than a third of the fat. What's more, the salmon offers a crowd of omega-3 benefits, and the cukes offer a few grams of fiber.

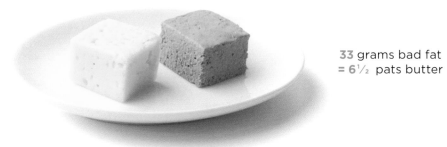

33 grams bad fat
= 6½ pats butter

1 ½-ounce cube havarti cheese **170 calories** **14 grams fat**
1 ½-ounce cube liver pâté **205 calories** **19 grams fat**

TOTAL **375** calories **33** grams fat

VS.

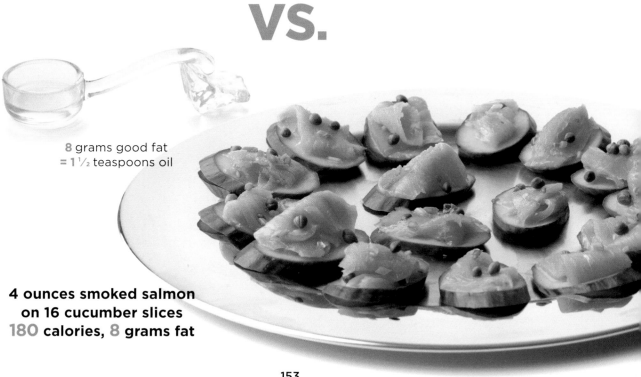

8 grams good fat
= 1 ½ teaspoons oil

**4 ounces smoked salmon
on 16 cucumber slices
180 calories, 8 grams fat**

OOH LA LA!

The French have a word for it, of course. And that single cup of genuine French onion soup looks pretty *petit* next to those mountainous bowls of *moules meunières*—mussels steamed with herbs, shallots and wine. At about a quarter of the calories and less than half the fat, the three bowls of mussels are a much better deal than the onion soup—just as delicious and far better for you. *Formidable!*

1 cup French onion soup
450 calories, 34 grams fat

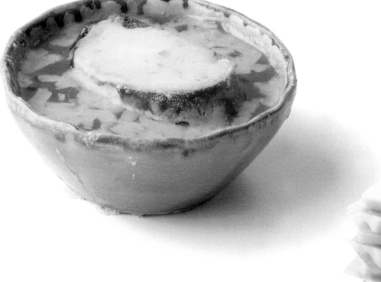

VS.

34 grams bad fat
= 7 pats butter

1 pound mussels cooked
with wine, herbs and garlic
150 calories, 3 grams fat
(x 3 = 450 calories, 9 grams fat)

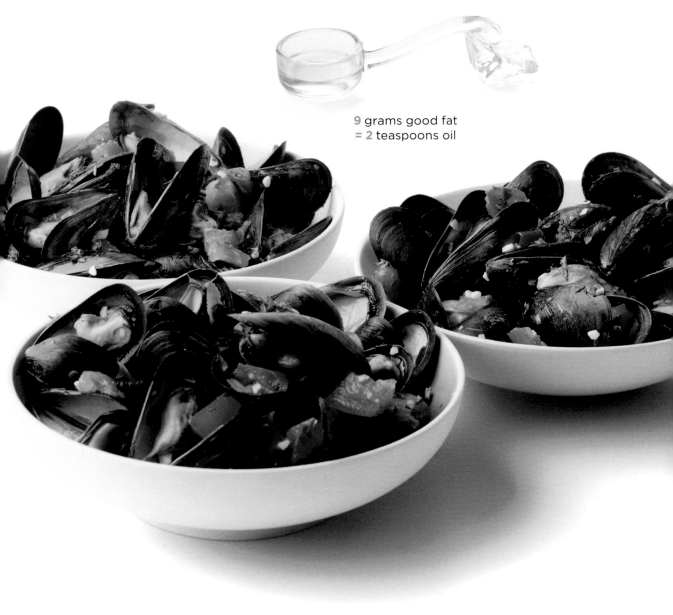

9 grams good fat
= 2 teaspoons oil

A GREAT RECIPE FOR A HEALTHY SOUP

Here's a recipe for a wonderful soup that is truly healthy and oh so satisfying.

COLD TOMATO AND AVOCADO SOUP

2 pounds ripe tomatoes

1 medium European or Kirby cucumber, peeled, halved and seeded

1 large garlic clove

$^3/_4$ cup chilled tomato juice

2 tablespoons lemon juice

1 tablespoon extra-virgin olive oil

$^1/_2$ teaspoon salt

$^1/_4$ teaspoon freshly ground black pepper

$^1/_2$ ripe avocado, cut into $^1/_4$-inch chunks

1 $^1/_2$ tablespoons slivered fresh mint leaves

1. Bring a medium saucepan of water to a boil over high heat. Place a tomato in the pan and boil for 30 seconds to loosen the skin. Cool under cold running water and slip off the skin. Repeat with the remaining tomatoes.

2. Core the tomatoes and cut into quarters. With your fingers, scrape out the tomato seeds and discard.

3. In a food processor or blender, working in batches if necessary, process the tomatoes, cucumber and garlic until very smooth. Place in a bowl and stir in the tomato juice, lemon juice, oil, salt and pepper. Cover and chill for at least 1 hour, or until ready to serve.

4. In a small bowl, gently combine the avocado and mint.

5. Ladle the soup into four serving bowls. Evenly divide the avocado mixture among the bowls.

Yield: 4 servings

Per serving: 140 calories, 8 grams fat

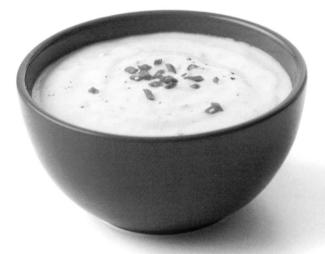

VS.

1 cup vichyssoise
320 calories, 29 grams fat

Cold Tomato and
Avocado Soup
140 calories, 8 grams fat

SHRIMP FOR DINNER

Hungry for shrimp? Have a small cup of shrimp fried rice and take in 26 grams of the bad kind of fat. Or down two bowls of this soup with shrimp. The latter is a satisfying main course that gives you the added nutritional power of varied vegetables, the good kind of fat and exceptional Creole-style taste.

CREOLE-STYLE RED BEAN SOUP WITH SHRIMP

1 tablespoon olive oil

6 scallions, thinly sliced

1 medium green bell pepper, chopped

1 rib celery, chopped

2 cups vegetable broth

1 15½-ounce can red kidney beans

1 14-ounce can Italian-style tomatoes, chopped

½ teaspoon marjoram, crushed

½ teaspoon freshly ground black pepper

12 ounces medium shrimp, peeled and deveined, tails left on

1. Heat the oil in a Dutch oven over medium heat. Add the scallions, bell pepper and celery and cook, stirring frequently, for 4 minutes, or until the vegetables are tender, adding some of the broth, 1 tablespoon at a time, if the pan gets dry.

2. Stir in the beans with their liquid, tomatoes with their juice, marjoram, black pepper and the remaining broth. Bring to a boil over high heat. Reduce the heat to low, cover and simmer, stirring occasionally, for 15 minutes, or until the flavors have blended.

3. Add the shrimp and cook, uncovered, stirring frequently, for 2 minutes, or until the shrimp are opaque.

Yield: 4 servings

Per serving: 210 calories, 5 grams fat

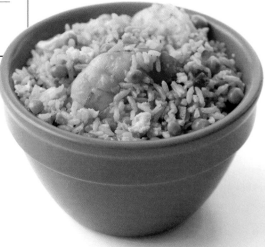

1 cup shrimp fried rice
420 calories, 26 grams fat

2 servings Creole-Style Red Bean Soup with Shrimp
420 calories
10 grams fat

MATCH POINT

Here comes the waiter with a tray of standard cocktail party pastry treats. And over there are three other cocktail party choices: shrimp with cocktail sauce, mouth-watering asparagus wrapped in veggie ham and grilled mushrooms in a black bean sauce. The food on all three groaning-board platters matches the calorie count of that modest tray of pastry hors d'oeuvres. But the savings in fat and the gain in nutrition from these seafood and vegetable delights are matchless.

2 ounces pastry-type hors d'oeuvres

(pigs-in-blankets, cheese straws, spanikopita, etc.)

270 calories, 18 grams fat

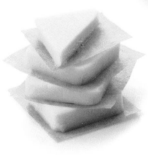

18 grams bad fat
= **3**½ pats butter

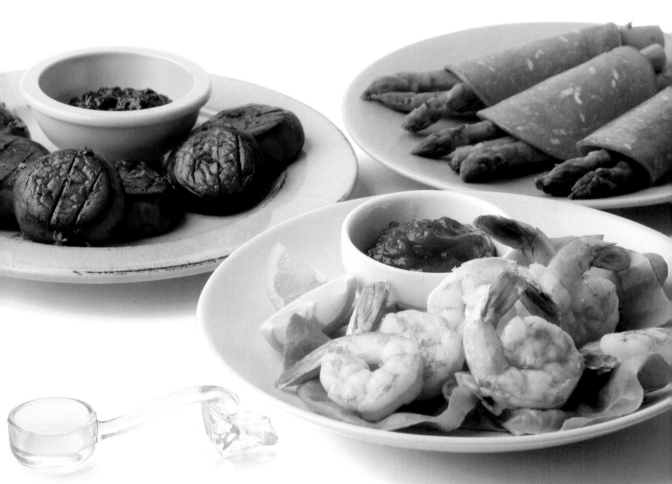

4 grams good fat
= 1 teaspoon oil

4 ounces shrimp 140 calories 2 grams fat
with cocktail sauce

9 stalks marinated asparagus 80 calories 1 gram fat
wrapped in 3 slices veggie ham

6 grilled mushrooms 50 calories 1 gram fat
with 2 tablespoons black bean sauce

TOTAL **270** calories **4 grams fat**

ITALIAN FEAST

If you love the taste of Italian sausage and peppers, take a look at these two virtually identical platters. Same amount of food, same delicious taste. But now note the difference in calories and fat content. That's where the resemblance ends.

4 ounces Italian sausage	382 **calories**	31 **grams fat**
1 ½ cups sautéed peppers	85 **calories**	3 **grams fat**
TOTAL	467 calories	34 grams fat

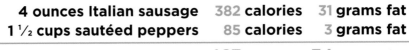

VS.

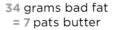

34 grams bad fat
= 7 pats butter

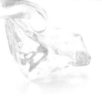

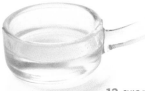

12 grams good fat
= **2** ½ teaspoons oil

4 ounces veggie Italian sausage	**186** calories	**9** grams fat
1½ cups sautéed peppers	**85** calories	**3** grams fat
TOTAL	**271** calories	**12** grams fat

DO THE MATH

A picture may be worth a thousand words, but even a Picture Perfect demo may not speak as eloquently as the numbers in this food comparison. On your left is a fairly uninteresting, only mildly appetizing meal of braised beef and plain white rice. On your right, a multicolored, multitaste, multitextured meal of foods right off the Beat Diabetes Pyramid: fish, fresh vegetables and yummy sautéed portobello mushrooms. Just check out the numbers: that small, dull dinner comes in at nearly three times the calorie count of the Pyramid meal and with nearly five times the fat.

VS.

34 grams bad fat
= 7 pats butter

2 4-ounce slices braised beef brisket	**600 calories**	**34 grams fat**
2 cups plain white rice	**440 calories**	**0 grams fat**
TOTAL	**1,040** calories	**34** grams fat

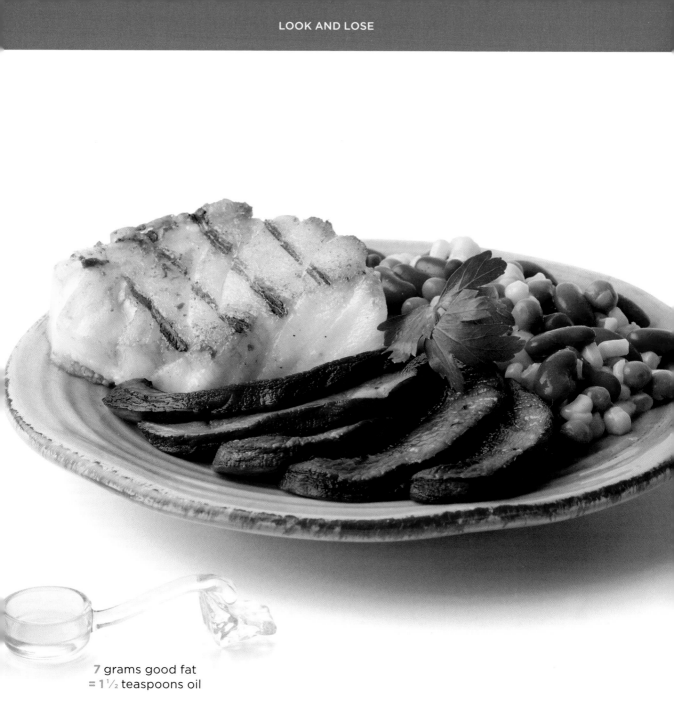

7 grams good fat
= 1 ½ teaspoons oil

6 ounces grilled fish (any white fish) 180 **calories** 2 **grams fat**
1 cup beans, peas and corn 160 **calories** 0 **grams fat**
1 cup sliced portobello mushrooms, sautéed 60 **calories** 5 **grams fat**

TOTAL **400** calories **7** grams fat

CHINESE CHOICES

Each of these three typical Chinese meals offers an appetizer from Column A and a main dish from Column B, but just look at the differences among them in calories and fat. Just about anyone interested in weight loss and diabetes prevention would eschew the first meal with its fried egg roll and high-fat meat choice. True, the middle choice saves you considerable calories and fat while adding some fiber and nutrition, but it's still fairly high in refined carbohydrates. The final choice is all Pyramid. With vegetable wonton soup, full-flavored seafood and mixed veggies in ginger sauce and healthful brown rice, it's a complete and very tasty arsenal of weight-loss and diabetes-fighting weapons.

Egg roll	405 **calories**	19 **grams fat**	2 **grams fiber**
6 ounces orange beef	460 **calories**	24 **grams fat**	0 **grams fiber**
1 cup pork fried rice	440 **calories**	20 **grams fat**	1 **gram fiber**
TOTAL	**1,305** calories	**63** grams fat	**3** grams fiber

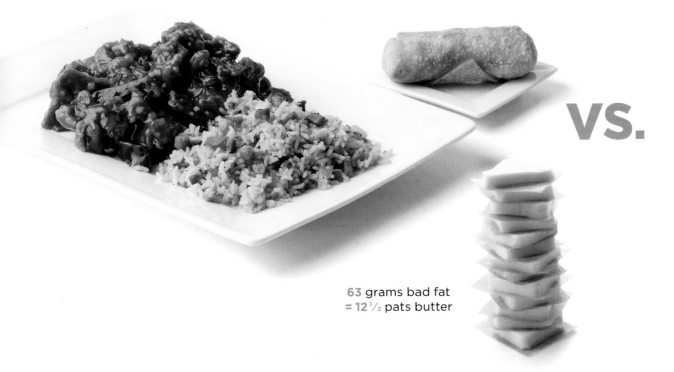

VS.

63 grams bad fat
= 12 ½ pats butter

4 steamed vegetable dumplings	240 calories	1 gram fat	2 grams fiber
6 ounces chicken, 2 cups Chinese vegetables in ginger sauce	400 calories	14 grams fat	10 grams fiber
1 cup steamed white rice	220 calories	0 grams fat	0 grams fiber
TOTAL	860 calories	15 grams fat	12 grams fiber

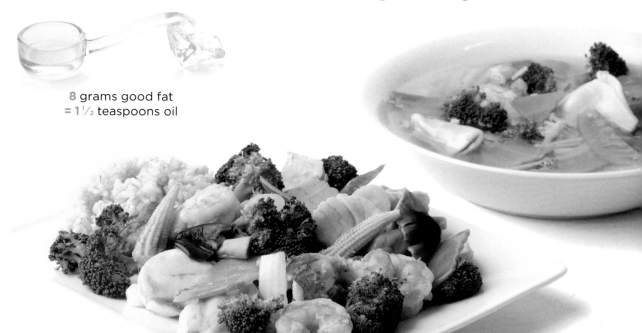

15 grams bad fat
= 3 pats butter

or

1 ½ cups vegetable wonton soup	80 calories	1 gram fat	4 grams fiber
6 ounces assorted seafood, 2 cups Chinese vegetables in ginger sauce	290 calories	7 grams fat	10 grams fiber
½ cup brown rice	110 calories	0 grams fat	2 grams fiber
TOTAL	480 calories	8 grams fat	16 grams fiber

8 grams good fat
= 1 ½ teaspoons oil

BARBECUE

Summertime means barbecue to many, but how will you do it this summer? Here's a meager barbecue on the left: a single sausage, a single burger and a single piece of buttered garlic bread—and just look at the tally of calories and fat! Contrast it with this groaning board of barbecued items—veggie sausage and burger; shrimp and peppers grilled on a skewer; corn, mushrooms and onion. Not to mention a healthy slice of watermelon for dessert. All of it comes in at way less than half the calories of that meager choice on the left, with one tenth the fat, and it has the added plus of fiber to help you keep the weight off and fight diabetes. In fact, with every bite, you're eating the Pyramid way and gaining health.

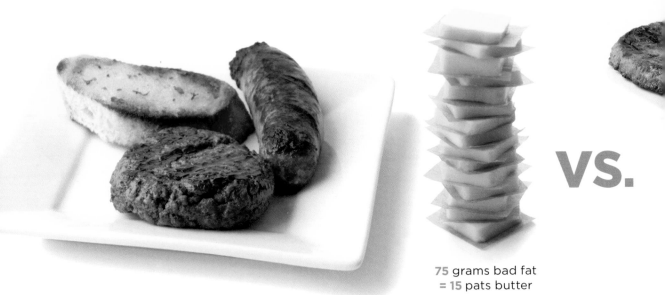

VS.

75 grams bad fat
= 15 pats butter

1 sausage, 3 ½ ounces	350 **calories**	30 **grams fat**	0 **grams fiber**
1 burger, 3 ½ ounces	290 **calories**	21 **grams fat**	0 **grams fiber**
3 ounces garlic bread	240 **calories**	0 **grams fat**	0 **grams fiber**
1-ounce butter	220 **calories**	24 **grams fat**	0 **grams fiber**
Garlic	0 **calories**	0 **grams fat**	0 **grams fiber**
TOTAL	**1,100** calories	**75** grams fat	**0** grams fiber

6 grams good fat
= 1 ½ teaspoons oil

1 veggie sausage, 3 ½ ounces	**150 calories**	**5 grams fat**	**2 grams fiber**
1 veggie burger, 2 ½ ounces	**70 calories**	**½ gram fat**	**4 grams fiber**
4 large shrimp and ½ pepper	**40 calories**	**½ gram fat**	**1 gram fiber**
1 ear corn	**120 calories**	**0 grams fat**	**2 grams fiber**
2 portobello mushrooms	**30 calories**	**0 grams fat**	**2½ grams fiber**
2 slices red onion	**30 calories**	**0 grams fat**	**1½ grams fiber**
1 slice watermelon (1 pound)	**50 calories**	**0 grams fat**	**1 gram fiber**
TOTAL	**490 calories**	**6 grams fat**	**14 grams fiber**

LESS PASTA, JUST AS MUCH TASTE

You love pasta, but as this bowl of pasta in cream sauce on the left seems to confirm, you're sure your waistline and your health would be better off if you stopped eating it. You don't have to. Here's a way of getting your hit of pasta taste by eating just half the amount of pasta but the same amount of food. And check out the savings in calories in fat—plus the added fiber this choice provides.

Pasta with cream sauce

4 ounces pasta	**420** calories	**0** grams fat	**0** grams fiber
1 cup cream sauce (e.g., Alfredo, vodka)	**590** calories	**54** grams fat	**0** grams fiber
TOTAL	**1,010** calories	**54** grams fat	**0** grams fiber

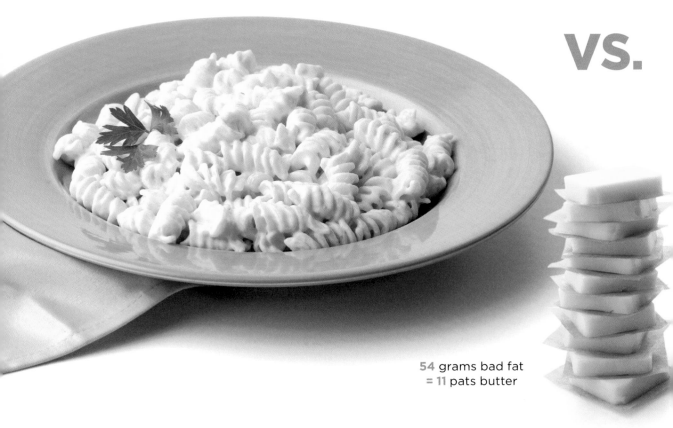

VS.

54 grams bad fat
= 11 pats butter

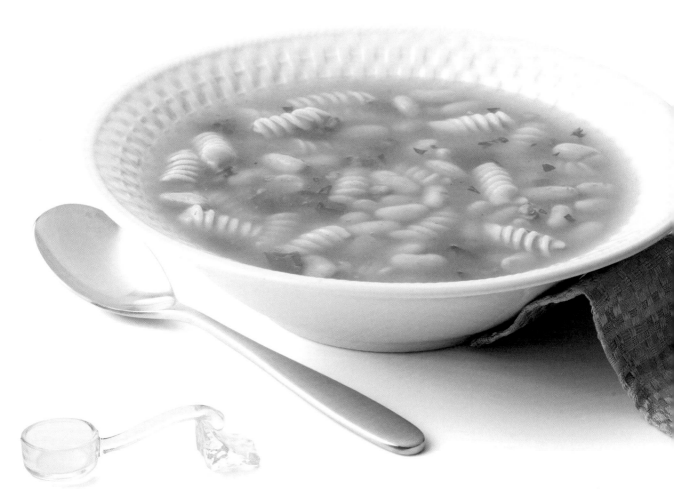

1 gram good fat
= 0 teaspoons oil

Pasta e fagiole

2 ounces pasta	210 calories	0 grams fat	0 grams fiber
1 cup broth	20 calories	1 gram fat	0 grams fiber
1 cup beans	230 calories	0 grams fat	15 grams fiber
TOTAL	460 calories	1 gram fat	15 grams fiber

LESS PASTA, EVEN MORE TASTE

Don't want to give up the taste of pasta in meat sauce? We don't blame you—and here's a way to enjoy not just that taste but a whole Pyramid of tastes. In addition to the pasta-in-meat-sauce taste that you love, you'll also get delicious zucchini in tomato sauce, a superb soup of white beans and spinach, and the meaty taste of marinated mushrooms on greens. Even with all that food, your tally is fewer calories and half the fat of the pasta in meat sauce alone, plus 17 grams of fiber for nutrition.

Pasta with meat sauce

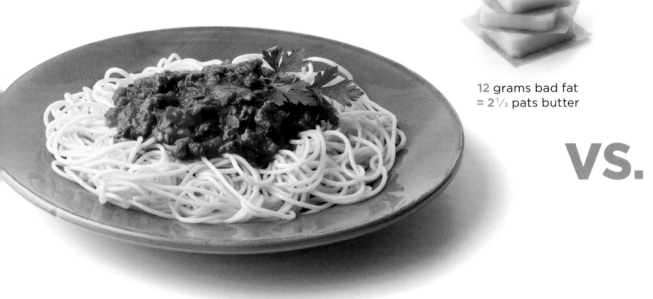

12 grams bad fat
= 2 1/2 pats butter

VS.

4 ounces pasta	**420 calories**	**0 grams fat**	**0 grams fiber**
1 cup meat sauce	**280 calories**	**12 grams fat**	**1 gram fiber**
TOTAL	**700** calories	**12** grams fat	**1** gram fiber

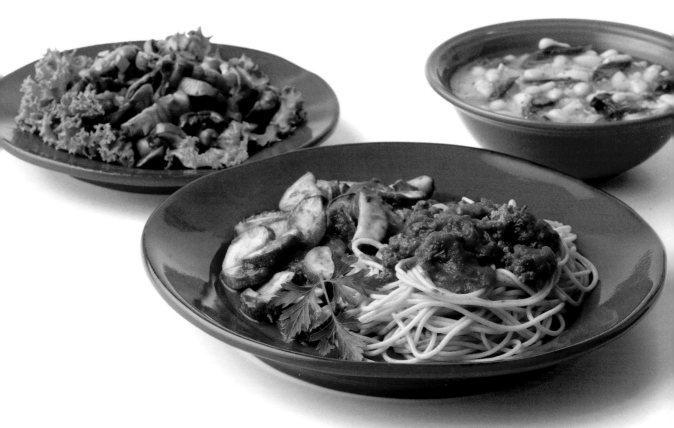

6 grams good fat
= 1 teaspoon oil

2 ounces pasta	210 calories	0 grams fat	0 grams fiber
½ cup veggie sauce	70 calories	2 grams fat	2 grams fiber
1 cup zucchini in tomato sauce	50 calories	1 gram fat	3 grams fiber
1 ½ cups white bean and spinach soup	180 calories	2 grams fat	10 grams fiber
1 cup marinated mushrooms on greens	20 calories	1 gram fat	2 grams fiber
TOTAL	**530** calories	**6** grams fat	**17** grams fiber

HOW MANY SKEWERS?

How many skewers of kebabs can you eat? One? Two? More? This single skewer of lamb kebab costs as many calories—and has four times as much fat!—as all four of these scallop-and-mushroom kebabs. Eat one, two, three or more of these tasty and healthful skewers and fight diabetes in the bargain.

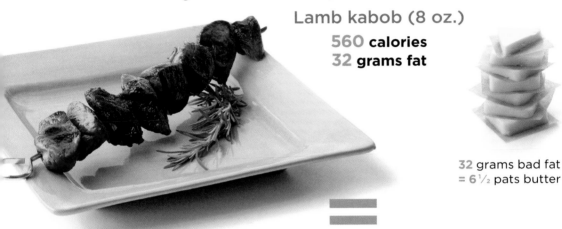

Lamb kabob (8 oz.)
560 calories
32 grams fat

32 grams bad fat
= 6 ½ pats butter

=

4 scallop-and-mushroom kabobs
(each with 4 oz. scallops, 4 oz. mushrooms and teriyaki sauce)
560 calories, 4 grams fat

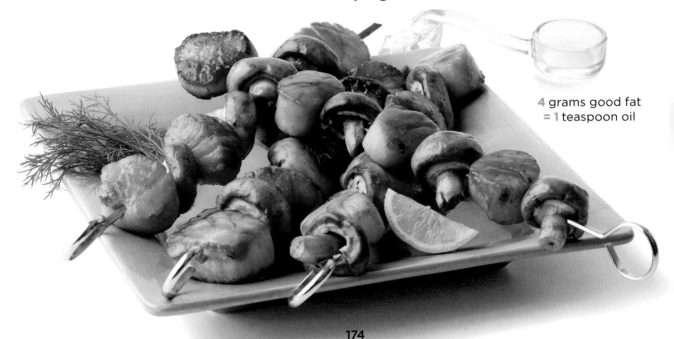

4 grams good fat
= 1 teaspoon oil

GOOD FOR YOU

The raspberry tart looks small and insignificant, and it has fruit, so it must be good for you, right? Well, take a look at the amount of calories, fat and sugar it contains. There's a better way to enjoy the sweetness of raspberries, as shown in this generous serving—and you add the benefits of phytonutrients as well.

Raspberry tart
320 calories, 15 grams fat

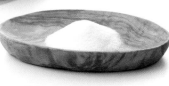

15 grams bad fat
= 3 pats butter

7 teaspoons sugar

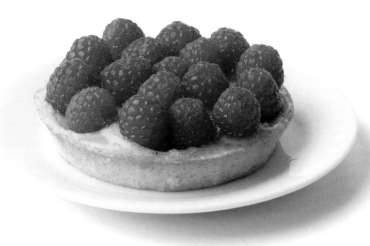

VS.

1½ cups red and black raspberries with a small amount of whipped topping

80 calories
9 grams fiber

DESSERT CHOICES

It isn't just the high calorie count and fat content of the rugelach that make them a tough choice if you're trying to lose weight and fight diabetes. It's also the added sugar! Neither the dried fruit nor the fresh fruit has any added sugar, nor any fat, of course. So if your choice is a platter of pastry or the generous serving of dried fruit shown here, go for the dried fruit. Or fix yourself a mountain of fresh fruit to save even more calories.

4 rugelach
480 calories, 24 grams fat

VS.

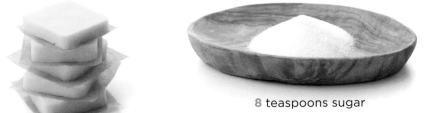

24 grams bad fat
= 5 pats butter

8 teaspoons sugar

5 dried apricots 100 **calories**
3 prunes 70 **calories**
2 dried pear halves 60 **calories**

TOTAL **230** calories

0 added sugar

0 pats butter

or

½ pound grapes 110 **calories**
1 small pear 40 **calories**

TOTAL **150** calories

0 added sugar

0 pats butter

SUGAR ADDED

Not all dried fruit products are equal. In some cases, the manufacturers add sugar, as in this cup of mixed berries, pineapple and papaya. Be sure to check the package to see if you might be taking in more sugar than needed. You'll see the calorie difference between the sweetened dried fruit and the unsweetened as well.

1 cup sweetened, mixed dried fruit
(berries, pineapple and papaya)
360 calories

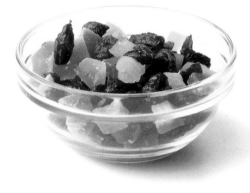

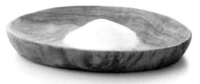

5 teaspoons added sugar

3 dried peach halves 60 **calories**
5 black mission figs 100 **calories**
3 dried apricot halves 30 **calories**

TOTAL 190 **calories**

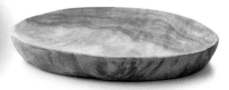

0 added sugar

CHOCOLATE BIG OR SMALL

How will you take your chocolate? In small bits that cost you big-time in calories and fat? Or in large mouthfuls that minimize the calories, have no fat at all and actually add the benefits of phytonutrients?

Chef Franklin suggests you try making your own chocolate dip for fruit by melting no-sugar-added chocolate bars.

2 truffles, ½ ounce each 140 **calories** 9 **grams fat**

3 pieces chocolate-covered 195 **calories** 10 **grams fat**
creams, nougats, etc.
(1½ ounces total)

TOTAL 335 **calories** 19 **grams fat**

VS.

5 large chocolate-covered strawberries
150 **calories,** 2 **grams fat**

LONG-LASTING SWEETNESS

It's true: all candies have pretty much the same amount of sugar per ounce, and this Tootsie Pop is pure sugar. But it is only 60 calories of sugar, equivalent to the amount of sugar in half an apple. What's more, while we tend to consume these mini chocolate chips almost mindlessly— by the handful, barely savoring the taste while taking in lots of calories and fat—a Tootsie Pop is a treat we can enjoy for a while. And once it's done, we don't need to reach for another and another and another...

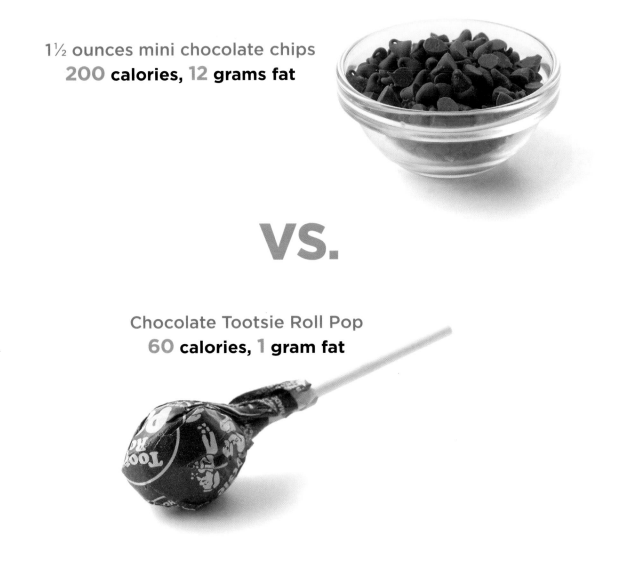

1½ ounces mini chocolate chips
200 calories, 12 grams fat

VS.

Chocolate Tootsie Roll Pop
60 calories, 1 gram fat

ICE CREAM BY THE NUMBERS

How much do you love the taste of ice cream? And how much ice cream do you want? The numbers here tell the story: this single scoop will cost you dearly in calories, fat and sugar. Or you could have seventeen of these no-sugar-added fudge pops and frozen fruit bars.

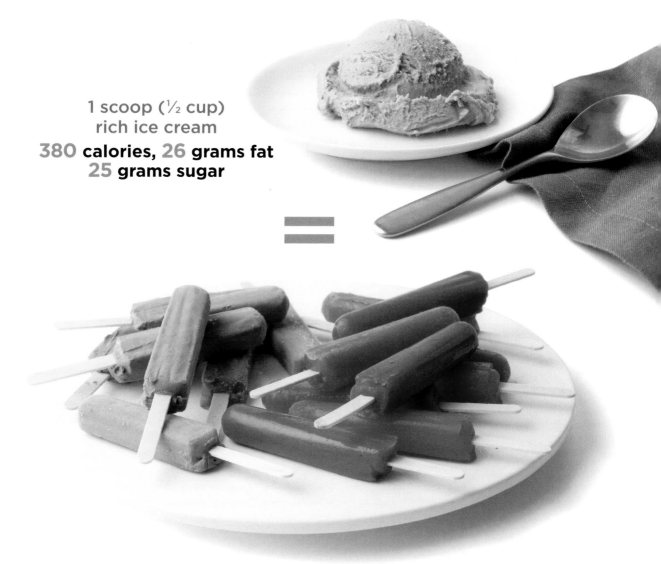

1 scoop (½ cup)
rich ice cream
**380 calories, 26 grams fat
25 grams sugar**

=

17 no-added-sugar fudge pops
and frozen fruit bars
380 calories

181

SABOTEURS

Saboteur foods come in many forms and are found everywhere. Where weight loss and diabetes prevention are issues, it's important to look beyond the packaging.

WHAT'S IN A MUFFIN?

This Fiber One muffin contains just about everything the health-conscious muffin lover looks for. Just read the package: Whole grains! Wild blueberries and oats! A whopping 28 percent of the Daily Value of fiber! All at one-fourth fewer calories than the leading muffin! So what could possibly be bad about making this muffin the core of your breakfast or an afternoon snack?

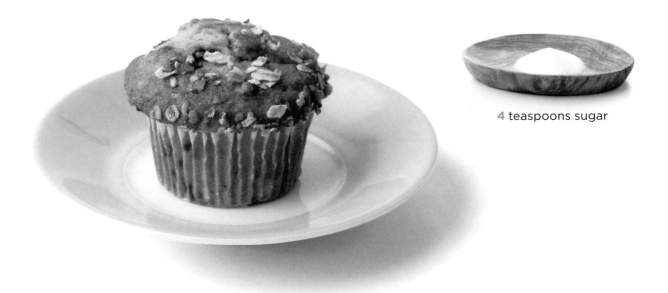

4 teaspoons sugar

How about the 16 grams of sugar in every single muffin? That's 4 teaspoons of sugar— just what you want to avoid if you're trying to maintain a healthy weight and fight diabetes. Especially if you eat two or three.

SUGAR-FREE?

"Sugar-free" is the way these oatmeal cookies are described, and sugar-free is what they are. Okay, but each serving—and a serving is just three cookies—contains 14 grams of starch from flour. And since starch is metabolically equivalent to sugar, there's no difference where your waistline and your health are concerned. That's why you're seeing 4 teaspoons of starch.

What's more, the fat contained in sugar-free cookies is very often the saturated fat that can seriously undermine your attempts to maintain a healthy weight and fight diabetes. This serving, for example, contains 7 grams of fat. That's why sugar-free cookies tend to be saboteur foods: because they're free of sugar, we allow ourselves to eat more of them—and end up taking in starch and fat!

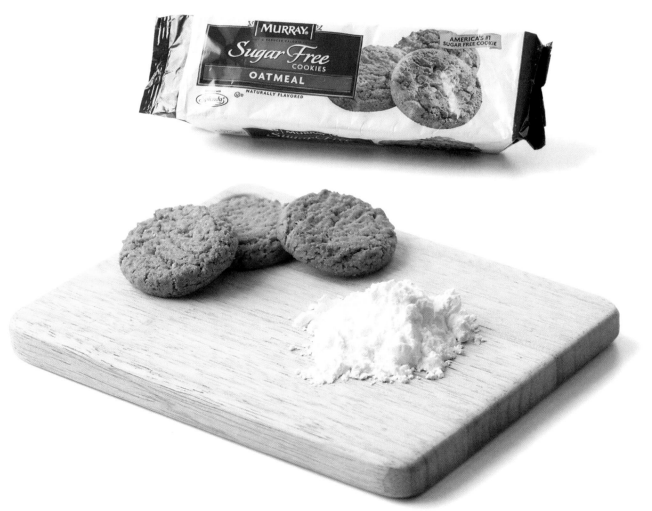

WATCH OUT FOR LOW-FAT PRODUCTS!

Weight Watchers is as reputable a program as there is, and its products are equally reputable. But as this demonstration makes clear, even with Weight Watchers, you can sometimes rationalize the situation and sabotage your own weight-loss effort.

This Weight Watchers Giant Fudge Bar rates only a single point on the Weight Watchers program, so it sounds like a food that's appropriate for anyone interested in weight loss—until you note that it contains 16 grams of sugar, represented here by the 4 brimming teaspoons of sugar on the plate.

Here's a better idea: when you crave a lush dessert, go for the many choices available on the Beat Diabetes Pyramid. They have no sugar at all. That makes them not just low-fat but downright good for your waistline, good for the fight against diabetes and still good-tasting.

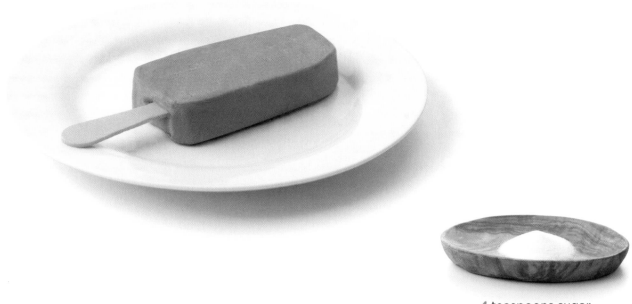

4 teaspoons sugar

CHAPTER 10

Recipes for Beating Diabetes

Here are recipes from Chef Franklin Becker and some of his celebrated colleagues—executive chefs from major restaurants around the country. Of course, all the recipes constitute eating the Beat Diabetes Pyramid way.

FRANKLIN BECKER RECIPES

THREE-BEAN SALAD WITH GINGER-LEMON VINAIGRETTE

The flavors of spring abound in this light, colorful salad. While it makes a fine first course on its own, you can also serve it as a side dish with a number of fish entrées.

1 cup snow pea pods

1 cup sugar snap peas

1 cup haricots verts

½ cup red cherry tomatoes, halved

½ cup yellow cherry tomatoes, halved

¼ cup snow pea shoots

¼ cup basil leaves

2 tablespoons finely minced ginger

¼ cup fresh lemon juice (1 to 2 lemons)

1 tablespoon Champagne vinegar or white wine vinegar

¼ cup extra-virgin olive oil

1 tablespoon honey

Kosher salt

Freshly milled white pepper

1. **Blanch the snow pea pods, sugar snap peas and haricots verts separately in boiling salted water until only slightly crunchy, 2 to 3 minutes; immediately shock each batch in an ice water bath to stop the cooking process and maintain their bright green color.**

2. **Remove the beans from the water when cooled, and dry them off with paper towels or a clean dish towel. Toss the beans together with the tomatoes and set aside.**

3. **Gently combine the pea shoots and basil together in a separate bowl, and refrigerate until they are ready to use to prevent them from wilting.**

4. **For the dressing, whisk together the ginger, lemon juice, vinegar, olive oil and honey, and season with salt and pepper to taste.**

5. **Dress the beans lightly with the vinaigrette, and the basil and shoots even more lightly to maintain their texture and avoid the addition of excess fat (from the oil) in your diet. Combine together after dressing.**

NOTE: The slightly sweet Champagne vinegar is a favorite of many chefs, but white wine vinegar is easier to find and will work just as well for this recipe.

VARIATION: Whenever possible, I recommend using locally grown vegetables for maximum flavor and freshness. So if any of the ingredients called for in this recipe are not in season, feel free to substitute something that is; for example, you can replace the snow pea shoots with a handful of mesclun greens.

Yield: 8 servings

CUCUMBER-MANGO SALAD

8 beefsteak tomatoes

1 tablespoon red wine vinegar

Kosher salt

Freshly milled white pepper

2 English cucumbers, medium dice

1 cup halved cherry tomatoes

1 red onion, small dice

1 mango, peeled, medium dice

½ cup fresh basil, chiffonade

1 tablespoon extra-virgin olive oil

To turn this salad appetizer into a larger meal, serve it with seafood, such as grilled shrimp, soft-shell crabs or raw oysters.

1. Cut the beefsteak tomatoes in half across, and place them in a microwave-safe casserole dish. Microwave the tomatoes on high for 4 minutes.

2. Remove the tomatoes, and use the back of a large spoon to gently press them through a strainer to make "tomato water."

3. Stir the tomato water together with the vinegar, and season with salt and pepper to taste. Set aside until ready to use.

4. In a mixing bowl, combine the cucumbers with the cherry tomatoes, onion, mango and basil, and season with salt and pepper to taste.

5. Place the salad in the center of a large bowl. Pour enough tomato water around the salad to come approximately halfway up the sides. Drizzle the salad lightly with olive oil and serve.

NOTE: If you do not own a microwave, the beefsteak tomatoes can be prepared using a large sauté pan. Cut the tomatoes in half across, and place them cut side down in the pan in a single layer. Turn the heat on low and cook the tomatoes until they soften and begin to lose their shape, approximately 10 to 15 minutes.

Yield: 8 servings

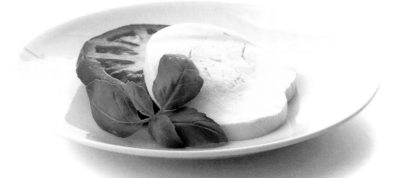

**Sliced tomato and mozzarella cheese (approx. 1½ ounces)
140 calories**

2 servings (2 cups)
of Cucumber-
Mango Salad
140 calories

VEGETABLE STOCK

½ bunch flat-leaf parsley

1 sprig thyme

1 bay leaf

15 black peppercorns

2 tablespoons canola oil

5 celery stalks, chopped

1 white onion, chopped

2 carrots, chopped

3 leeks, white parts only, chopped

1 large fennel bulb, chopped

1 garlic head, halved across

Vegetarian chefs have long known that vegetable stock is a great way to flavor soups and sauces without the addition of any meat products. In addition, it is filled with vitamins and other important nutrients. I actually prefer using vegetable stock over chicken stock when preparing lighter soups and sauces.

1. Make a sachet with the parsley, thyme, bay leaf and peppercorns. Heat a Dutch oven on low; add the canola oil and sauté the celery, onion, carrots, leeks and fennel until they begin to soften, approximately 10 minutes. Add 4 quarts of cold water, garlic and the sachet, and simmer for 1 hour.

2. Strain and cool down the liquid. This stock can be refrigerated for up to 5 days, or frozen in pint containers for up to 2 months.

Yield: 16 cups

MUSHROOM LENTIL SOUP

1 tablespoon grapeseed oil

1 tablespoon chopped onion

2 teaspoons chopped celery

2 teaspoons chopped carrot

2 garlic cloves, chopped

15 to 20 white button mushrooms, chopped (2 cups)

1 cup green or brown lentils

Mushroom stock (see below)

1 tablespoon crème fraîche

1 teaspoon kosher salt

½ teaspoon freshly milled black pepper

Cooked French green lentils hold their shape well, making them a good choice for this soup. Brown lentils may be substituted, however, as they are usually easier to find in supermarkets.

1. In a saucepot over medium heat, heat the grapeseed oil and then add the onion, celery, carrot and garlic. Cook until the vegetables are tender but not brown, approximately 4 minutes, lowering heat if necessary.

2. Add the mushrooms, lentils and stock. Cover the pot and simmer until the lentils are tender but not mushy, approximately 30 minutes.

3. Remove the mixture from the pot and transfer to a blender. Add the crème fraîche, salt and pepper, and process until smooth. Taste the mixture, and add additional seasoning if necessary.

NOTE: Before using lentils in a recipe, it is important to rinse them well and check closely for pebbles with your fingers.

Yield: 8 servings

MUSHROOM STOCK

2 tablespoons grapeseed oil

1 onion, chopped

2 celery stalks, chopped

1 carrot, chopped

2 garlic cloves, chopped

25 to 30 white button mushrooms, chopped (3 cups)

1 bunch thyme

1. In a Dutch oven over medium heat, heat the grapeseed oil. Add onion, celery and carrots, and cook until the onion becomes translucent, approximately 4 minutes (stir occasionally to keep the vegetables from browning).

2. Add the garlic, mushrooms and thyme, and continue cooking and stirring to soften the vegetables, an additional 15 minutes.

3. Cover the vegetables with 2 quarts of cold water, bring just to a boil and simmer uncovered for 30 minutes.

4. Turn off the heat and allow the ingredients to sit in the pot for 30 minutes more. Pour the mushroom stock through a fine mesh strainer, and discard the solids.

VARIATION: This stock can be made with just about any mushrooms you have available, although different types will produce different flavors.

CAULIFLOWER ALMOND PUREE

2 heads cauliflower

1 garlic clove, chopped

1 leek, white part only, cleaned and chopped

2 tablespoons olive oil

½ cup almonds, toasted

2 tablespoons almond oil

¼ cup crème fraîche

1 teaspoon kosher salt

½ teaspoon freshly milled white pepper

A key ingredient in this recipe is almond oil, available at most gourmet retailers and some online food Web sites. Nut oils, including almond oil, walnut oil, hazelnut oil and pistachio oil, are monounsaturated, helping raise desired HDL cholesterol and lower "bad" LDL cholesterol...and they taste great, too.

1. **Cut off the thick stem from the cauliflower and discard. Separate the cauliflower heads into individual florets with your hands or a knife, and rinse under cold water to clean.**

2. **Place the cauliflower, garlic, leeks and olive oil in a Dutch oven, and add 2 cups of water. Bring to a boil, and then turn down to a simmer. Cook vegetables until fork-tender, about 30 minutes. Drain the vegetables over a bowl, reserving the liquid for later use.**

3. **Add the vegetables to a blender, along with the toasted almonds, almond oil and crème fraîche, and process until smooth. Season with salt and pepper, and adjust the consistency using the reserved liquid until the desired consistency is achieved.**

NOTE: **To toast almonds or almost any dried nuts, place on a baking sheet in an oven or toaster oven in a single layer, and cook at 350°F until golden brown, approximately 10 minutes. Shake the tray periodically to avoid uneven cooking, and check the nuts often to make sure they do not burn.**

Alternatively, you can cook the almonds in a dry sauté pan on medium heat, tossing them every minute or so to ensure even browning.

Yield: 4 servings

STEAMED MUSSELS HOTPOT WITH SAKE BROTH

1 tablespoon bonito flakes

1 sheet kombu, rinsed

2 cups water

1 cup light soy sauce

½ cup sake

2 tablespoons sweet cooking rice wine

2 tablespoons unsalted butter

1 pound Prince Edward Island mussels, cleaned

2 tablespoons chopped lemongrass

2 tablespoons chopped fresh ginger

1 tablespoon grated fresh ginger

2½ cups sake broth

2 tablespoons chopped scallions, green parts only

Kosher salt

Freshly milled white pepper

Prince Edward Island (PEI) mussels, which are far less expensive than clams, oysters or shrimp, are one of my favorite varieties. Imported New Zealand mussels are also excellent and have an attractive green shell, but they normally cost more than PEI mussels and can be harder to find.

BROTH

1. Slowly bring all of the sake broth ingredients to a simmer (be sure not to boil the broth, or it will become cloudy). Simmer for 20 minutes, and then remove from heat. Let the broth steep off the heat for another 20 minutes before straining through a piece of cheesecloth.

MUSSELS

1. To clean the mussels, soak them briefly in cold water to remove any grit; mussels with shells that remain open after cleaning are dead and should be discarded. Just before using the mussels, rip out the inedible "beard" (a tangle of threads that sticks out of the shell).

2. Melt 1 tablespoon butter in a large sauté pan. Add the mussels and toss to coat. Add the lemongrass, ginger and sake broth, and simmer, covered, until the mussels open, approximately 4 minutes.

3. Add the scallions and the remaining butter, season with salt and pepper to taste and serve hot.

Yield: 2 servings

GRILLED CALAMARI WITH MEDITERRANEAN CUCUMBER SALAD

12 calamari, tubes and tentacles

9 tablespoons extra-virgin olive oil

2 sprigs rosemary

2 sprigs thyme

2 shallots, chopped

2 tablespoons red wine vinegar

1 teaspoon kosher salt

½ teaspoon freshly milled white pepper

2 medium tomatoes, seeded

1 English cucumber, peeled and seeded

3 tablespoons chopped basil

½ teaspoon red pepper flakes

Calamari (squid) is very inexpensive—especially when compared with the cost of shrimp or scallops—and, like any other seafood, it is high in protein and low in fat.

1. Marinate the calamari tubes and tentacles with 3 tablespoons olive oil, rosemary, thyme and shallots in the refrigerator for 3 to 4 hours before cooking.

2. To make the vinaigrette, combine 6 tablespoons olive oil and the vinegar in a bowl, and season with salt and pepper.

3. For the Mediterranean cucumber salad, cut the tomatoes and cucumbers into medium dice. Toss the tomatoes, cucumber, basil and red pepper flakes together with the vinaigrette.

4. Season the calamari lightly with salt and pepper, and grill at medium heat on a grill pan or outdoor barbecue until opaque, 1 to 2 minutes per side (be careful not to overcook the calamari, or they will become tough and rubbery).

5. Spoon the cucumber-tomato salad onto a plate, and place the grilled calamari around the salad. Pour some of the remaining vinaigrette over the calamari.

VARIATION: A combination of grilled scallops, shrimp or a mixture of these plus the calamari will work well for this dish. In addition, frozen calamari may be used in place of fresh in this recipe.

Yield: 4 servings

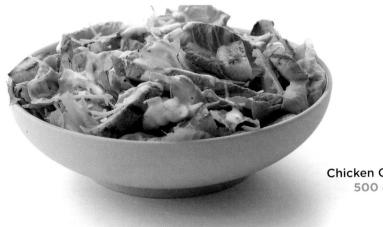

Chicken Caesar Salad
500 calories

2 servings (2 cups)
Grilled Calamari
with Mediterranean
Cucumber Salad
500 calories

GRILLED SHRIMP WITH SHAVED FENNEL

15 jumbo shrimp, peeled and deveined

9 tablespoons extra-virgin olive oil

2 sprigs rosemary

2 sprigs thyme

2 shallots, chopped

1 tablespoon white wine vinegar

1 tablespoon fresh lemon juice

1 tablespoon fresh lime juice

3 oranges, segmented, plus 1 tablespoon fresh orange juice

1 teaspoon kosher salt

½ teaspoon freshly milled black pepper

2 fennel bulbs, shaved thin

Chiffonade ½ bunch mint leaves

I created this dish while working as the chef of a popular restaurant in Brooklyn. It employs the basic philosophy of Italian cooking: use the freshest ingredients possible, and let their natural flavors shine through clearly. Here, the licorice taste of the fennel, combined with mint and citrus, brightens and enhances the shrimp.

1. Marinate the shrimp with 3 tablespoons olive oil, rosemary, thyme and shallots in a bowl for approximately 1 hour in the refrigerator.

2. To make the shaved fennel, combine 6 tablespoons extra-virgin olive oil and vinegar with the lemon juice, lime juice and orange juice in a separate bowl, and season with salt and pepper. Add the orange segments, fennel and mint.

3. Season lightly with salt and pepper and grill at medium heat on a grill pan or outdoor barbecue until cooked through, approximately 2 minutes per side.

4. To serve, place the shaved fennel in the center of the plate, reserving the liquid. Place the shrimp on top, and drizzle the liquid around the plate.

VARIATION: The shrimp can also be prepared in a sauté pan on medium heat until cooked through, approximately 2 minutes per side.

Yield: 5 appetizer servings

QUINOA LINGUINI WITH WHITE CLAM SAUCE

1 dozen littleneck clams

1 dozen Manila clams

1 dozen cockles

3 tablespoons extra-virgin olive oil

Kosher salt

8 ounces quinoa linguini (or any other whole-grain pasta)

1 small onion, diced

3 garlic cloves, minced

½ cup white wine

1 8-ounce can clam juice

½ bunch flat-leaf parsley, chopped

Freshly milled white pepper

While this recipe calls for littleneck clams, Manila clams and cockles, it is fine to use only littleneck clams if the others are unavailable. Cherrystone clams may also be substituted without any loss of flavor, but they will be chewier.

1. Scrub the clamshells well with a brush and rinse under cold water to remove any grit.

2. Bring 1 gallon water to a boil in a large pot. Add 1 tablespoon of olive oil and 1 tablespoon salt to the water. Add the pasta and cook until just al dente, approximately 10 minutes, and then strain through a colander.

3. While the pasta is cooking, heat 2 tablespoons olive oil in a large pan. Add all the littleneck clams, Manila clams and cockles to the pan. Add the onion and garlic and toss everything together.

4. Slowly pour in the wine and bring to a boil. Add the clam juice and return the liquid to a boil; cover the pan until the clams and cockles open, approximately 2 to 4 minutes.

5. Remove and reserve the clams and cockles in their shells and return any remaining liquid to the pan.

6. Add the pasta to the broth and cook 2 minutes longer. Add the clams, butter (if using) and parsley to the pan just before serving, and season with salt and pepper to taste.

VARIATION: To make your own clam juice at home, purchase 6 to 8 chowder clams, scrub the shells thoroughly with a brush and steam them in a pot with ¼ cup water until they open, approximately 10 minutes. Discard the shells and strain the juice through a fine-mesh strainer wrapped with cheesecloth to remove any remaining grit. The chowder clams may be chopped up and added to the dish, if desired.

Yield: 4 servings

RED SNAPPER IN TOMATO-SAFFRON BROTH

Artichoke Oreganata Puree
(see opposite page)

10 plum tomatoes

1 cup tomato juice

1 garlic clove, smashed

1 tablespoon saffron

Kosher salt

Freshly milled white pepper

3 tablespoons extra-virgin
olive oil

6 6-ounce red snapper
fillets, skin on

Saffron may be the most expensive spice, but it usually only requires a few pinches to flavor a dish, and the results are always impressive. Saffron is the stigma of a certain type of crocus, and these stigmas must be picked by hand and then dried before packaging. No wonder it's so expensive!

1. **For the tomato broth, cut the tomatoes into quarters lengthwise and scoop out the seeds with a knife; discard the seeds. Puree the tomatoes in a blender, and then add the tomato juice and 1 cup water.**

2. **Pour the puree into a pot and add garlic, saffron and salt and pepper to taste. Bring the mixture to a boil, and then transfer to a clear plastic container.**

3. **Cool the liquid until it begins to separate. Slowly strain through a fine-mesh strainer, reserving the liquid.**

4. **Heat a stainless steel sauté pan on medium-high until very hot, approximately 5 minutes. Pour the olive oil into the pan; immediately add the red snapper fillets, skin side down. Cook until the bottom of the fish begins to curl up around the edges, approximately 5 minutes. Turn the fish over and continue cooking until the flesh is opaque throughout, about 2 minutes more.**

5. **To serve, place a dollop of the artichoke oreganata puree in the center of the bowl. Spoon some broth around the bowl, and place the fish on top.**

VARIATION: **Red snapper is one of the more common fish available today in most parts of the United States, but other fish that will work just as well in this dish include black sea bass and striped bass.**

Yield: 6 servings

1 tablespoon canola oil

½ tablespoon chopped onion

1 teaspoon chopped celery

1 teaspoon chopped carrot

1 garlic clove, chopped

1 cup fresh artichoke bottoms (2 to 3 artichokes), or 1 cup frozen artichoke hearts

1 lemon

¼ cup white wine

¼ cup vegetable stock

2 teaspoons white wine vinegar

1 teaspoon sour cream, or 1 tablespoon low-fat sour cream

1 teaspoon kosher salt

¼ teaspoon freshly milled black pepper

¼ cup dried Italian seasoned bread crumbs

ARTICHOKE OREGANATA PUREE

1. Warm a sauté pan on medium heat for approximately 3 minutes. Add the canola oil and then the onion, celery, carrot and garlic. Cook until tender but not brown, about 10 minutes, lowering the heat if necessary.

2. To prepare fresh artichoke bottoms (if using), follow these steps:

   a. To prevent the artichokes from browning, fill a bowl with cold water, and squeeze the juice from the lemons into the bowl. Prepare the artichoke bottoms one at a time, placing each one in the lemon water as soon as they are trimmed.

   b. Cut off the stem of the artichoke, followed by the top of the leaves above the heart.

   c. Snap off the outer leaves, and use a paring knife to remove the remaining leaves.

   d. Cut the artichoke bottom in half, and scoop out the hairy inner choke with a small spoon and discard.

3. Add the fresh artichoke bottoms to the pan, if using, and continue cooking until completely tender, approximately 10 minutes more. (If using frozen artichoke hearts, add them to the pan at this point and cook until hot, approximately 5 minutes.)

4. Deglaze with white wine. Add stock and vinegar and simmer until most of the liquid in the pan has evaporated, around 5 minutes. Remove the mixture from the pan and transfer to a blender along with sour cream, salt, pepper and bread crumbs. Blend and serve beneath red snapper.

SESAME TOFU AND VEGETABLE STIR-FRY

1 tablespoon canola oil

1 tablespoon minced ginger

2 garlic cloves, minced

2 bunches scallions, green parts only, julienne

2 cups snow pea pods

2 cups baby bok choy, sliced

1 cup mung bean sprouts

1 8-ounce can water chestnuts

1 15-ounce package firm tofu, large dice

1 teaspoon toasted sesame seeds

1 teaspoon toasted sesame oil

Kosher salt

Freshly milled white pepper

Stir-frying in a wok or sauté pan is a great way to cook vegetables quickly with a small amount of oil. It also helps retain necessary vitamins and minerals, as well as the freshness of the vegetables.

1. **Heat a wok or large sauté pan on medium-high for 5 minutes. Add the canola oil, and then the ginger, garlic and scallions.**

2. **Add the vegetables at approximately 30-second intervals, beginning with the snow pea pods, and followed by the bok choy, mung bean sprouts and water chestnuts. Add the tofu, and cook until the snow pea pods are tender, 3 to 4 minutes total.**

3. **Add the sesame seeds and sesame oil, and season with salt and pepper to taste. Serve immediately to maintain the crispness of the snow pea pods and bok choy.**

NOTE: **Tofu is packed with protein, calcium and iron and is low in fat, making this dish a great vegetarian entrée for lunch or dinner.**

Yield: 8 servings

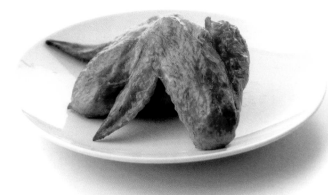

2 chicken wings
230 calories

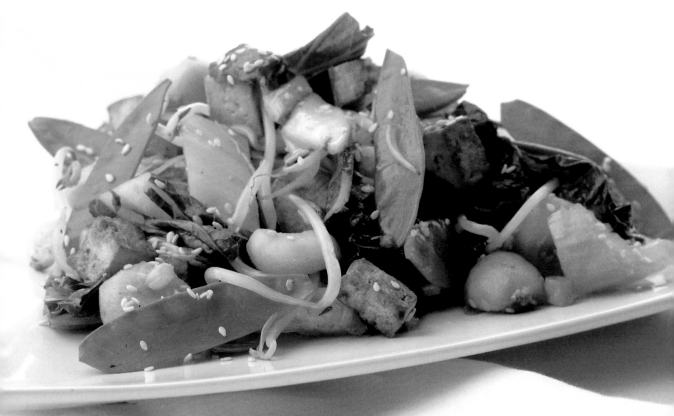

1 serving Sesame
Tofu and Vegetable
Stir-Fry
230 calories

GRILLED HALIBUT AND BUCKWHEAT SALAD

½ cup uncooked buckwheat

2 cups string beans, diced

4 medium tomatoes, diced

1 bunch flat-leaf parsley, chopped

2 bunches scallions, green parts only, chopped (1⅓ cups)

Chiffonade ½ bunch mint

¼ cup fresh lemon juice (1 to 2 lemons)

Kosher salt

Freshly milled white pepper

8 6-ounce halibut fillets

½ cup extra-virgin olive oil

Parsley for garnish

Roasted buckwheat (kasha) is commonly used in Eastern European cooking. It is treated as a grain and can be cooled after cooking and mixed with vegetables and other ingredients to form a nutritious salad like the one used in this dish.

1. Bring 1 cup water to a boil. Stir in the buckwheat, cover tightly and simmer on very low heat until the buckwheat becomes tender and all the liquid is absorbed, approximately 6 to 8 minutes.

2. Allow the buckwheat to cool, and then toss together with the string beans, tomatoes, parsley, scallions, mint, lemon juice and olive oil to make the salad. Season with salt and pepper to taste.

3. Brush the halibut lightly with olive oil and season with salt and pepper. Grill on a grill pan or outdoor barbecue, or sauté on both sides over medium heat, until cooked through, approximately 4 minutes per side.

4. To serve, place the fish on top of the salad. Garnish with parsley.

VARIATION: An equal amount of wheat berries may be used in place of buckwheat in this recipe. Both buckwheat and wheat berries are great sources of fiber.

Yield: 8 servings

OLIVE OIL POACHED HALIBUT WITH BRAISED FENNEL

1 cup extra-virgin olive oil

1 tablespoon fresh lemon juice

1 tablespoon white wine vinegar

1 fennel bulb, small dice

1 yellow onion, small dice

¼ cup brine-cured black olives

1 sprig thyme

1 medium tomato, diced

Kosher salt

Freshly milled white pepper

4 6-ounce halibut fillets

1 lemon

The method of poaching fish in olive oil is far healthier than it might sound. Firm fish such as halibut will not soak up much oil during poaching; and as long as it is dabbed dry with a paper towel after cooking, there will be no more oil than if the fish were sautéed. Poaching in olive oil also ensures that the fish will remain moist and flavorful.

1. For the braised fennel, preheat oven to 350°F. Combine the olive oil, lemon juice, vinegar, fennel, onion, olives and thyme in a baking dish, and cook in the oven until the fennel becomes soft, approximately 1 hour. Add the tomatoes, and season with salt and pepper to taste.

2. Strain the leftover olive oil from the fennel and reserve. Set aside the vegetables in a warm spot while preparing the fish.

3. Return the excess olive oil to the pot. Using a cooking thermometer to check the temperature of the oil (it should remain between 160°F and 180°F), poach the fish until cooked through, approximately 15 minutes. Remove the fish and pat off any excess oil with a paper towel.

4. To serve, spoon some of the braised fennel mixture onto a plate and place a halibut fillet on top. Garnish with a lemon wedge.

NOTE: Including the olives with the fennel early on will intensify the flavor of the dish; however, they may be added at any time during the cooking process.

NOTE: Kalamata, Gaeta and Niçoise are a few of the many types of brine-cured olives that will work well with this dish. It is fine to purchase pitted olives, but I would not recommend most canned or jarred olives, as I find that both the flavor and texture tend to be inferior.

Yield: 4 servings

BLACK SEA BASS WITH MEDITERRANEAN CUCUMBER-TOMATO SALAD

1 English cucumber, medium dice

2 medium tomatoes, medium dice

½ red onion, medium dice

¼ cup brine-cured black olives, pitted and chopped

Chiffonade ½ bunch mint

1 tablespoon red wine vinegar

4 tablespoons extra-virgin olive oil

½ teaspoon red pepper flakes

Kosher salt

Freshly milled white pepper

4 6-ounce black sea bass fillets

Additional mint for garnish (optional)

Salads with cucumber and tomatoes as the primary ingredients are very common in Mediterranean cooking. They are particularly enjoyable when ripe, flavorful tomatoes are used. The salad used in this dish is light, refreshing and healthy, making it an ideal summertime entrée.

1. For the salad, combine the cucumber, tomatoes, red onion, olives, mint, vinegar, olive oil and red pepper flakes, and mix together in a bowl. Season with salt and pepper to taste.

2. Brush the fish lightly with olive oil, sprinkle with salt and pepper and grill on a grill pan or outdoor barbecue until just cooked through, approximately 3 to 4 minutes per side.

3. To serve, spoon the salad onto a plate and place the grilled fish on top. Garnish with a chiffonade of mint, if desired.

VARIATION: Branzino, red snapper or halibut also go well with the cucumber-tomato salad in this recipe. The cooking method for each is the same.

Yield: 4 servings

MARINATED MUSHROOM ANTIPASTO

¼ cup extra-virgin olive oil

2 tablespoons red wine vinegar

1 teaspoon red pepper flakes

2 cups white button mushrooms, cleaned and quartered

1 cup cremini mushrooms, cleaned and quartered

Kosher salt

Freshly milled black pepper

2 tablespoons chopped flat-leaf parsley

These mushrooms are a good accompaniment to almost any entrée. Alternatively, they can be served as an appetizer in the summer, either by themselves or with other cold vegetables. One advantage to this dish is that it can be made up to three days ahead and refrigerated until ready to use.

1. Whisk together the olive oil, vinegar and red pepper to make a vinaigrette. Toss the mushrooms with half of the vinaigrette and set aside for 2 hours in the refrigerator to marinate.

2. Preheat the oven to 450°F. Transfer the mushrooms to a sheet pan and roast in the oven until browned, approximately 10 minutes. Remove the mushrooms from the oven and allow them to cool to room temperature.

3. Toss the roasted mushrooms together with the remaining vinaigrette, season with salt and pepper to taste and stir in the parsley just before serving.

NOTE: Cremini mushrooms are darker and have an earthier flavor than button mushrooms, but in appearance they are almost the same. If you are unable to find creminis, it is fine to use a total of 3 cups button mushrooms for this recipe.

Yield: 10 servings

BRUSSELS SPROUTS WITH MUSTARD SEEDS AND CURRY

1 tablespoon unsalted
clarified butter

1 tablespoon mustard seeds

1 teaspoon Madras curry
powder

Kosher salt

2 cups Brussels sprouts

Freshly milled white pepper

*For many of us, Brussels sprouts evoke childhood memories
of being told to "eat your vegetables, they're good for you."
While they are indeed nutritious, Brussels sprouts can also
taste wonderful—just be sure not to overcook them, which
can produce an unpleasantly strong flavor and smell.*

1. In a sauté pan, melt the clarified butter and add the
mustard seeds and curry. Turn off the heat and allow the
ingredients to sit for 10 minutes in the pan.

2. In a large pot, bring 1 gallon water to a rapid boil.
Add 3 tablespoons salt and return the water to a boil.
Add the Brussels sprouts and cook until just tender,
approximately 4 minutes. Drain in a colander.

3. Preheat the sauté pan on medium until the butter
begins to brown, and then add the Brussels sprouts.
Toss to coat, allowing the Brussels sprouts to brown
lightly. Season with salt and pepper to taste.

Yield: 4 servings

OKRA WITH SLOW COOKED ONIONS AND SPICY TOMATO SAUCE

1 cup homemade or store-bought tomato sauce

1 tablespoon red pepper flakes

2 ½ cups okra

1 lemon, juiced

¼ cup extra-virgin olive oil

4 yellow onions, large dice

4 garlic cloves, sliced

½ cup Gaeta, Kalamata or Niçoise olives

½ cup flat-leaf parsley, chopped

Kosher salt

Freshly milled white pepper

Okra is a popular ingredient in the South and is served in many different ways (probably the best known being gumbo). With a renewed interest in Southern cooking throughout the United States, okra has become more popular and easier to find in grocery stores in recent years.

1. Place the tomato sauce and red pepper flakes in a small pot and heat on low to a simmer. Turn off the heat, set aside and cover until ready to use.

2. Trim the ends off the okra and immediately place the okra in a bowl filled with cold water and the lemon juice to prevent them from browning.

3. Heat a sauté pan on medium for 3 minutes, add the olive oil and the onions and stir briefly. Reduce the heat to low and cook the onions until lightly caramelized, stirring often.

4. Add the garlic, olives, okra and tomato sauce and simmer until the okra becomes tender. Stir in the parsley and season with salt and pepper to taste.

Yield: 8 servings

STEWED RATATOUILLE

1 cup chopped tomatoes

1 tablespoon red pepper flakes

⅓ cup extra-virgin olive oil

1 onion, large dice

4 garlic cloves, sliced

1 red pepper, julienne

1 yellow pepper, julienne

3 zucchini, sliced

3 yellow squash, sliced

1 small eggplant, quartered and sliced across

½ cup Gaeta, Kalamata or Niçoise olives

1 bunch flat-leaf parsley, chopped

Kosher salt

Freshly milled white pepper

1. Place the tomatoes and red pepper flakes in a small pot and heat on low to a simmer. Turn off the heat, set aside and cover until ready to use.

2. Heat a sauté pan on medium and add 1 tablespoon olive oil. Sauté the onion and garlic together until the onions are translucent, approximately 3 minutes; remove and place in a large bowl.

3. Return the pan to the heat, add 2 tablespoons olive oil and sauté the red and yellow peppers for 4 minutes. Remove and add to the bowl with the onions and garlic.

4. Next, sauté the zucchini and yellow squash in 1 tablespoon olive oil until they begin to lose their firmness, approximately 3 minutes, and add to the bowl.

5. Finally, turn up the heat to medium-high; add 2 more tablespoons olive oil and sauté the eggplant until it begins to soften, approximately 2 minutes. Stir in the tomato sauce and olives, and pour the mixture into a pot.

6. Simmer the vegetables until they are very tender but not mushy, approximately 20 minutes. Add the parsley, and season with salt and pepper to taste.

VARIATION: The method for this recipe calls for sautéing all the vegetables separately to ensure none will overcook, but to save time you can also use the following technique. Pour all the olive oil into a hot pan (use two pans if necessary), followed by the onion and garlic; a minute later, add the peppers, a minute after that the zucchini and yellow squash, and finally the eggplant slices.

Sauté all the vegetables together until they begin to lose their crispness and the onions become translucent, an additional 2 to 3 minutes. Stir in the tomatoes and olives, and simmer until very tender, add parsley and season.

Yield: 8 servings

1 cup creamed spinach
360 calories

3 servings (3 cups)
Stewed Ratatouille
360 calories

GIARDINIERA (ITALIAN-STYLE PICKLED VEGETABLES)

1 pound kirby cucumbers, in pieces ½ inch long

1 pound celery stalks, in pieces ½ inch long

2 tablespoons pickling salt

1 head cauliflower, in pieces

2 carrots, peeled and cut into ½-inch-long pieces

1 pound cippolini onions or shallots

1 pound red peppers, seeded and cut into ½-inch lengths

½ pound garlic cloves

1 quart water

1 quart white wine vinegar

½ cup olive oil

3 bay leaves

2 teaspoons black peppercorns

3 sprigs thyme

3 sprigs oregano

1. Salt the cucumbers and celery for 2 hours with ½ tablespoon of the pickling salt. Drain and toss with remaining vegetables.

2. In a stainless-steel or other nonreactive pot, bring the vinegar, water and salt to a boil. Add the vegetables to the liquid and boil, covered, for 20 minutes. This will alleviate the need for refrigeration.

3. Combine the olive oil with the bay leaves, black peppercorns, thyme and oregano, and set aside.

4. Pack the vegetables evenly into hot, sterilized jars along with the garlic, olive oil mixture and some of the cooking liquid, and seal. The jars can then be stored in a cool dark place for up to 3 months. The longer the vegetables sit the more "pickled" they will be.

Yield: 20 servings

SUGAR-FREE PANNA COTTA

2 cups almond milk

2 cups soy yogurt

1 envelope unflavored gelatin

¼ cup Splenda

Vanilla bean (or 1 tablespoon vanilla extract)

Try serving this with fresh fruit such as berries or grapes.

1. Bring the almond milk to a simmer and add the yogurt. Remove from heat and mix well.

2. Sprinkle the gelatin on top of the yogurt mixture, and allow to dissolve. Add the Splenda and the vanilla and transfer to 12 cups. Allow to chill in the refrigerator for several hours.

Yield: 12 servings

PEANUT BUTTER CUPS

2 ounces Splenda

6 ounces fresh peanut butter

16 ounces dark chocolate, melted

1. Combine the Splenda and peanut butter.

2. Coat a chocolate mold tray with melted chocolate, chill for 10 minutes and then fill each cup with peanut butter mixture. Top with chocolate and chill again until set.

Yield: 24 peanut butter cups

CITRUS GRANITA

1 cup orange juice

1 cup lemon juice

1 cup grapefruit juice

½ cup Splenda

4 cups ice water

1. Bring juices to a simmer and add the Splenda; stir to dissolve. Add the ice water and then move to the freezer to cool.

2. Pour into a pan and place in the freezer. Chill for 2 hours, then begin scraping the ice with a fork every half hour until you have a granita consistency (very much like large crystals of ice).

Yield: 14 ½-cup servings

20 calories per serving

½-cup scoop regular granita
80 calories

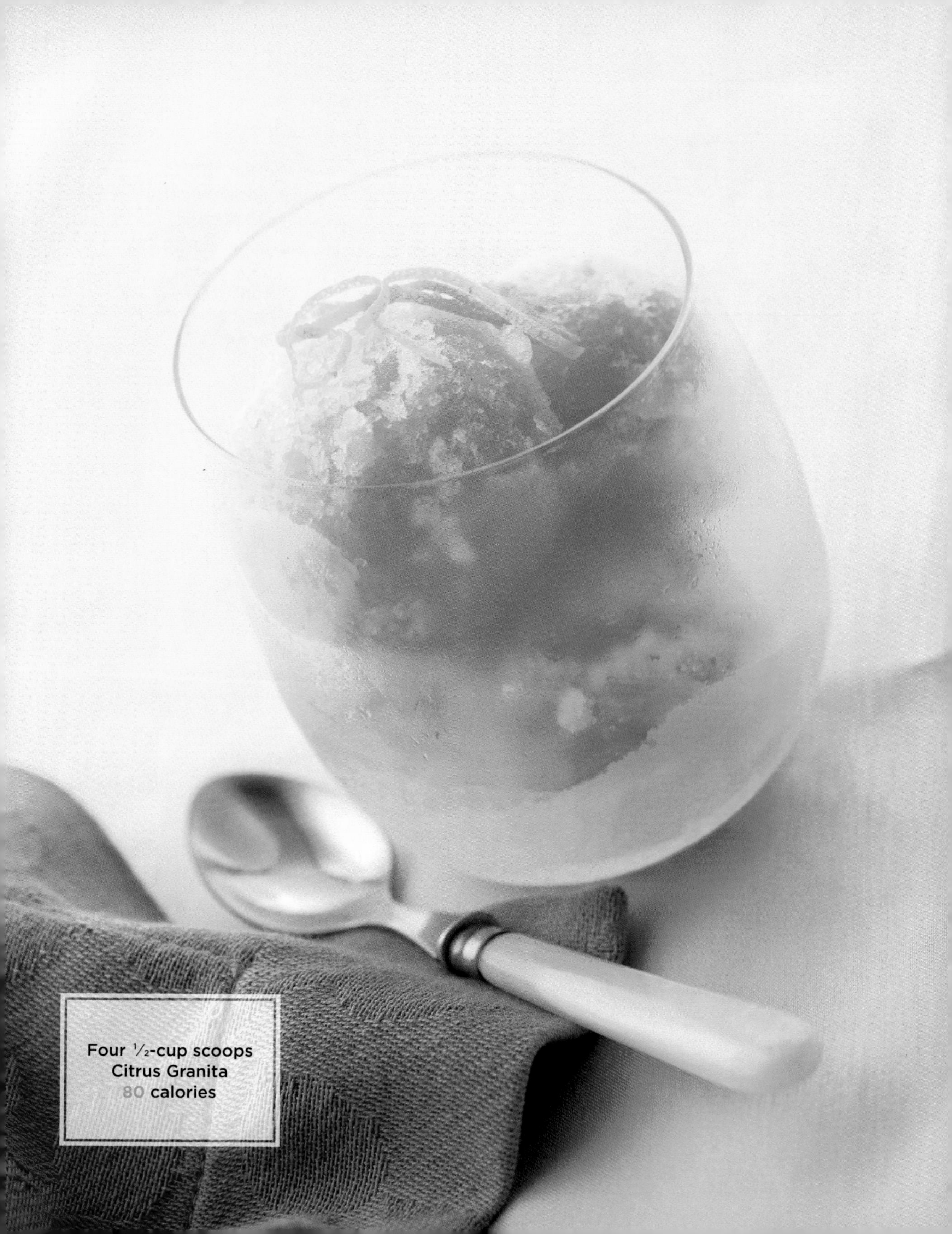

Four ½-cup scoops
Citrus Granita
80 calories

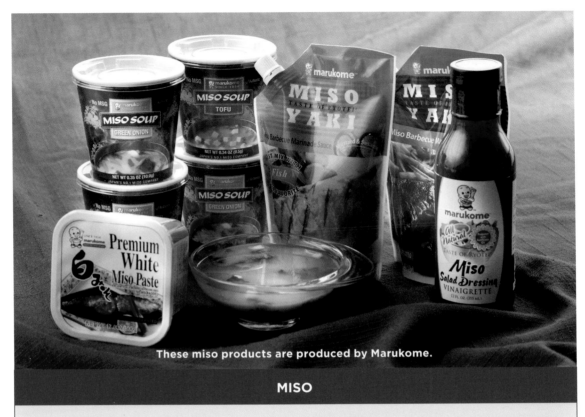

These miso products are produced by Marukome.

MISO

Soybean-based miso, the traditional seasoning of Japanese cuisine, is high in protein and rich in vitamins and minerals. Its use dates back to feudal Japan, and it is still widely consumed in both traditional and modern cooking—not just in its native land but worldwide as well. Deployed in a surprising range of dishes—pasta sauces, pizza toppings, salads, appetizers, fish and meat entrées, even refreshing sorbets and chocolates—the staple nevertheless remains miso soup. The traditional morning bowl has always been regarded by the Japanese as having cleansing and detoxifying qualities, and small wonder: miso soup is full of ingredients that contribute to good nutrition and health.

Miso's principal ingredient, the soybean, provides vital amino acids for our bodies. In addition, miso is an excellent source of iron, zinc, riboflavin and magnesium. Your cup of miso soup may cost as few as 36 calories.

With American interest in its properties and taste growing, it's no wonder that **Marukome, Japan's largest miso producer, has just built a state-of-the-art manufacturing facility in California to supply U.S. consumers with fresh miso—made from American ingredients.** In the picture above you can see many of the products they offer.

SHAVED CUCUMBER, RADISH AND ASIAN PEAR SALAD WITH MISO VINAIGRETTE DRESSING

2 English cucumbers, sliced thin

½ pound radishes, sliced thin

½ pound Asian pear, sliced thin

½ pound jicama, sliced thin

1 tablespoon scallions, sliced thin

1 tablespoon cilantro

¼ cup **Marukome brand** miso vinaigrette salad dressing

Salt

Pepper

1 lime, sliced into 6 pieces

1 tablespoon sesame seeds

1. Mix all of the fruit and vegetables and dress lightly with the dressing. Season with salt and pepper to taste. Serve with fresh lime wedges and a sprinkle of sesame seeds.

Yield: 6 servings

GLAZED SALMON WITH MISO YAKI MARINADE

1 ½ pounds salmon, skin off

1 teaspoon salt

2 tablespoons **Marukome miso yaki marinade**

1 teaspoon scallions, finely chopped

1 teaspoon red bell pepper, finely chopped

Serve this with salad or simply with a little steamed brown rice.

1. Season the salmon with salt and 1 tablespoon of the miso yaki marinade for 2 hours before cooking.

2. Heat the broiler and cook the salmon for 4 minutes before turning it over and glazing it with the remaining miso yaki marinade. Cook for 4 more minutes, garnish with scallions and red bell pepper.

Yield: 4 servings

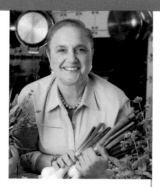

CELEBRITY CHEF RECIPES

Lidia Bastianich

Lidia Matticchio Bastianich is an award-winning chef, restaurateur, cookbook author and public television cooking show host. Her latest series, *Lidia's Italy,* was nominated for an Emmy in 2008 and named Best National Cooking Show by the James Beard Foundation in 2009. She is also the host of several earlier series and author of companion books, including *Lidia's Family Table, Lidia's Italian American Kitchen* and *Lidia's Italian Table.* Together with her daughter, Tanya, she wrote *Lidia Cooks from the Heart of Italy,* published in October 2009, along with another 52 episodes of *Lidia's Italy.*

In addition to over ten years with public television, Lidia is well known for her acclaimed restaurants, including the three-star Felidia and Del Posto restaurants in New York, the popular theater district restaurant Becco and the Lidia's restaurants in Kansas City and Pittsburgh. Lidia was named Outstanding Chef—U.S. and Outstanding Chef—New York by the prestigious James Beard Foundation.

Lidia and son Joseph Bastianich, well-known wine expert and restaurateur with multiple locations in New York, Las Vegas, Los Angeles and beyond, also produce award-winning wines at the Bastianich and La Mozza vineyards in Italy.

MUSSELS WITH FARRO, CANNELLINI AND CHICKPEAS

(FARRO, FAGIOLI, CECI E COZZE)

From *Lidia's Italy* (Knopf, 2007) As much as Puglia is about the land, it is also flanked by water: the Adriatic on one side and the Ionian Sea on the gulf side. Hence one finds a big tradition of seafood as one travels down to the tip of the heel.

In the quaint seaside city of Trani, along the Adriatic shoreline, is a delightful restaurant called Le Lampare. There I was introduced to *Farro con Legumi e Cozze,* a beautiful stew of ceci and cannellini beans cooked with farro, one of my favorite grains, tossed before serving with savory mussels and their juices.

1 cup dried chickpeas
1 cup dried cannellini beans
½ cup chopped carrots
½ cup chopped celery
1 cup chopped onion
1½ cups cherry tomatoes, cut in half
½ cup extra-virgin olive oil plus more for finishing
1 cup farro or pearled barley
1½ teaspoons coarse sea salt or kosher salt
½ teaspoon peperoncino
4 garlic cloves, crushed, peeled and sliced
2 pounds mussels
4 tablespoons chopped fresh Italian parsley

1. Rinse the chickpeas and place in a bowl with cold water, covering them by 4 inches. Do the same with the cannellini in a separate bowl. Soak both for 12 to 24 hours.

2. Drain and rinse the chickpeas and put them in a 5-quart heavy-bottomed saucepan with about 7 cups of fresh cold water. Set the pot over medium-high heat and drop in the chopped carrot, celery and onion, the halved cherry tomatoes, and 4 tablespoons of the olive oil. Bring the water to a boil, partially cover the pan and adjust the heat to maintain a steady, bubbling simmer. Stir occasionally.

3. After the chickpeas have cooked for an hour, drain and rinse the cannellini and stir them into the pot. There should be at least an inch of liquid covering the beans; add more water if necessary. Return to the boil, partially cover and simmer for 45 minutes, stirring now and then.

4. Rinse the farro grains in a sieve and stir in with the beans, along with the 1½ teaspoons salt and ¼ teaspoon of the peperoncino. There should be about ¼ inch of liquid covering the beans and grain; add more if necessary. Return to the boil, partially cover and simmer for about 30 minutes or longer, until the beans and the farro are tender—add water if needed to keep the beans and grains barely covered with liquid as they finish cooking. When they are done, most of the surface water should have been absorbed or evaporated but the stew should be slightly soupy.

5. While the farro cooks, prepare the mussels. Pour the remaining 4 tablespoons olive oil in a heavy 12-inch sauté pan, scatter in the garlic cloves and remaining ¼ teaspoon peperoncino. Cook for 3 minutes or so over medium-high heat, until the garlic is lightly colored, then add all the rinsed mussels at once. Tumble them around the pan quickly, to coat with oil and put on the cover. Cook over high heat for about 2 minutes, shaking the covered pan a couple of times, just until the mussels are open, and take the pan off the stove.

6. Shuck the mussels right over the pan, letting the juices and meat drop in. Discard the shells (and any mussels that did not open). If you like, leave a dozen or so mussels in the shell for a garnish.

7. When the farro and beans are cooked, pour the shucked mussels and their juices into the pot and stir well—the consistency should be rather brothy. Heat to the boil and cook for just a minute to make sure everything is nice and hot. Taste and adjust salt. Stir in the chopped parsley and spoon portions into warm pasta bowls; garnish with unshucked mussels if you saved them. Drizzle good olive oil over each and serve immediately.

To prepare in advance: Cook the beans and farro until tender, following recipe, and remove from the heat. Let them sit in the saucepan up to 3 hours (they will absorb liquid and thicken). Shortly before serving, cook and shuck the mussels. Stir the mussel juices into the beans and farro and heat slowly to a simmer. Stir in the mussels and finish as above.

Yield: 6 servings

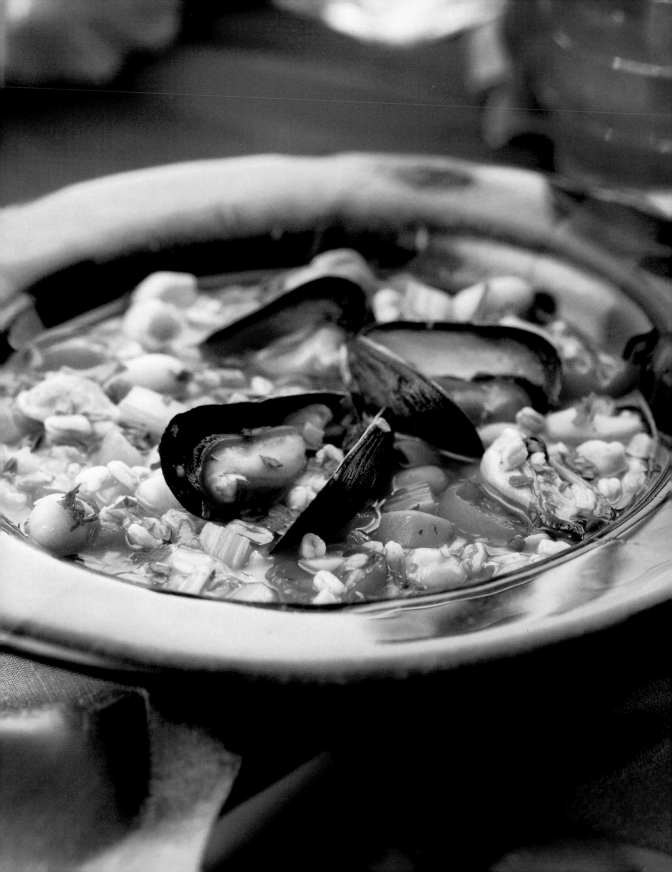

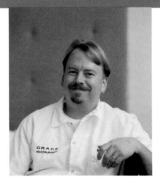

Neal Fraser

Neal Fraser began his culinary career in Los Angeles at the age of twenty, working as a line cook at Eureka Brewery and Restaurant, one of Wolfgang Puck's earliest restaurants. Inspired by this introduction to the life of a professional chef, Fraser entered the Culinary Institute of America in Hyde Park, New York. Fraser is now partner and executive chef at GRACE and serves his New American cuisine in an atmosphere perfectly designed to complement the ambitious flavors of one of Los Angeles' most revolutionary culinary talents.

SAUTÉED EUROPEAN SEA BASS WITH TOASTED COUSCOUS, ARTICHOKES, TOMATOES AND SAFFRON FENNEL BROTH

2 garlic cloves, minced

3 onions, chopped

1 stalk celery, chopped

1 head fennel, sliced

Olive oil

1 pinch saffron

1 vine-ripe tomato, seeded and chopped

1 cup white wine

Salt

2 cups lobster stock

2 ounces fresh basil, chopped

2 cups toasted couscous, preferably whole grain

4 medium to large artichokes

4 6-ounce fillets branzino (loup de mer) or other nice sea bass, skin on, pin bones removed

Pepper

1. **Heat the garlic, 1 onion, celery and fennel with 2 ounces olive oil until translucent. Add the saffron, tomato, half the white wine and salt to taste.**

2. **Reduce wine mixture by two-thirds, then add the lobster stock and basil and simmer for 1 hour. Strain and skim off any fat. Set broth to the side.**

3. **In a medium pot, heat 1 onion in 2 ounces olive oil until translucent. Add couscous and salt to taste and cover with water. Cook over medium heat until couscous is tender. Set to the side.**

4. **Peel artichokes to the choke and set aside in a bowl of water.**

5. **In a small sauté pot add the remaining white wine, 1 onion and 2 cups of water and bring to a boil.**

6. **Preheat oven to 400°F.**

7. **Boil for 10 minutes, then add artichokes along with salt to taste and simmer over medium flame until tender. Set to side.**

8. **Heat oven-safe sauté pan with 2 ounces olive oil. Season the fish with salt and pepper and place in pan skin side down.**

9. **Place in preheated oven for approximately 2–5 minutes, depending on the thickness of the fish.**

10. **Plate fish alongside couscous and artichokes; spoon on broth.**

Yield: 4 servings

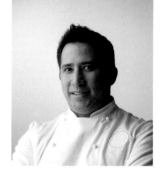

Christopher Lee

Christopher Lee was named among the "Top Ten Best New Chefs of 2006" by *Food & Wine* and "Best Chef 2005" by *Philadelphia* magazine as well as "Rising Star Chef of the Year" at the 2005 James Beard Awards. Lee became the executive chef for New York City restaurant Gilt in August 2006, where his cooking earned the restaurant two Michelin stars. Lee is currently the executive chef at Aureole in New York City.

CHILLED ENGLISH PEA SOUP WITH POACHED CANADIAN LOBSTER, BLOOD ORANGE, BABY PEA GREENS AND TARRAGON OIL

1 2-pound lobster

3 cups English peas, preferably fresh

3 shallots, peeled and sliced thin

2 garlic cloves, peeled and sliced thin

1 rib celery, sliced thin

4 cups water or vegetable stock

1 cup soy milk

Salt

Pepper

1 bundle tarragon

¼ cup vegetable oil

1 blood orange

¼ pound baby pea greens

1. Remove the tail and claws from the body of the lobster. Cook the tail for 5 minutes and the claws for 7 minutes in boiling water seasoned with salt. Immediately after cooking, shock the tails and claws in an ice bath. Once cooled, remove all the meat from the shells and cut into a medium dice. Reserve until serving.

2. Blanch the peas in boiling salted water until tender, about 4 minutes, then shock in an ice bath.

3. Heat a 6-quart pot over medium heat with 1 tablespoon vegetable oil and sweat the shallots, garlic and celery until tender. Then add the stock and cook for 25 minutes. Add soy milk and simmer for another 5 minutes. Allow to cool.

4. Once the base of the soup is cool add the blanched peas. Then blend the soup until smooth, pass through a fine strainer and season with salt and pepper. If the soup is a little too thick, thin it out with some water or soy milk. Refrigerate until serving.

5. Slice 2 tablespoons tarragon very thin and mix with 3 tablespoons vegetable oil. Combine with lobster and season with salt and pepper.

6. Peel the blood orange and cut into segments.

7. Using a small ring mold, make a nice mold of lobster salad in the middle of 4 bowls. Then pour the reserved soup around it and remove the mold. Place the blood orange segments on top of the lobster salad. Scatter the baby pea greens across the plate to finish.

Yield: 4 servings

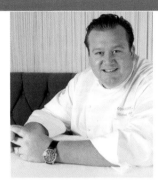

Michael White

Michael White became the executive chef at Fiamma Osteria in New York City in 2002. The restaurant garnered a glowing three-star review from the *New York Times* and White was named *Esquire*'s Best New Chef of that year. White then published the cookbook *Fiamma: The Essence of Contemporary Italian Cooking* in 2006. After helming the kitchen at a number of other successful Manhattan restaurants, White opened Marea in May 2009 and received yet another overwhelmingly positive three-star review from the *New York Times*.

TUSCAN BEAN SOUP WITH KALE AND SPELT

3 cups barlotti or cranberry beans, or substitute pinto beans

1 cup farro (spelt) or wheat berries

¼ cup extra-virgin olive oil, plus extra for drizzling

1 pound kale, preferably Tuscan, coarse stems removed, cut into thick ribbons (about 4 cups)

1 medium-large yellow onion, diced

1 large rib celery, trimmed and diced

3 garlic cloves, thinly sliced

5 cups vegetable stock

1 cup peeled, seeded and diced tomatoes

1 sprig rosemary

1 sprig sage

Sea salt

Freshly ground pepper

¼ cup freshly grated Parmigiano-Reggiano

1. In separate bowls, cover the beans and faro with cold water and soak overnight. Drain and carefully pick through them to remove any pebbles or foreign matter. Set aside.

2. In a large heavy pot, heat the olive oil over medium-high heat. Stir in the kale, onion, carrot, celery and garlic and cook, stirring occasionally, until the vegetables are softened, about 10 minutes.

3. Add the beans, farro, stock and tomatoes and bring the liquid to a boil.

4. Stir in the rosemary and sage, adjust the heat down so the liquid is simmering, and cook for 1 hour to 1 hour 10 minutes, until the beans are tender.

5. If the soup is too thick, stir in additional vegetable stock as needed. Season to taste with salt and pepper.

6. Ladle the soup into large bowls, drizzle with extra-virgin olive oil, sprinkle with Parmigiano-Reggiano cheese and serve immediately.

Yield: 6 servings

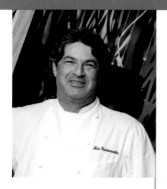

Kim Canteenwalla

Chef Kim Canteenwalla brings twenty-five years of culinary expertise as president of Blau and Associates, a highly successful restaurant consulting firm with a client list that includes top hospitality establishments.

Most recently, Canteenwalla joined forces with Steve Wynn to open Society Café Encore as executive chef/partner at the new signature resort in the Wynn collection. The restaurant offers guests a classic American menu of old-school favorites with a modern twist. Open for breakfast, lunch and dinner and late into the night on weekends, Society Café Encore features enjoyable food in a casual, fun and dynamic atmosphere.

He began his culinary career in Montreal at the Institute of St. Denis. He continued to work in his native Canada as sous-chef for the luxury five-star Four Seasons Hotel in Toronto. He then went on to serve in executive chef positions that took him all over the world, including Raffles International Hotel Group; Hotel Le Royal Phnom Penh, Cambodia; and Grand Mirage Resort Bali, Indonesia.

Upon his return to North America, Chef Canteenwalla held the position of executive chef at Beau Rivage, where he met Elizabeth Blau. He was then recruited to serve as executive chef for the MGM Grand Hotel and Casino in Las Vegas.

Canteenwalla was invited to prepare a guest chef dinner and lecture to the graduate students at the internationally famed Swiss Ecole Hotelière in Lausanne, Switzerland. In 2005, Canteenwalla teamed up with chef and partner Kerry Simon for the Food Network's *Iron Chef America* series and came home victorious.

NANTUCKET BAY SCALLOPS

6 ounces raw beluga lentils

2 bay leaves

2 garlic cloves, crushed

8 ounces turkey bacon

3 ounces butter

3 ounces olive oil

4 ounces shallots, finely chopped

6 ounces zucchini, skin on, finely chopped

6 ounces yellow squash, skin on, finely chopped

4 ounces green beans, chopped fine

Kosher salt

Coarse black pepper

10-12 ounces (approximately 32-40 pieces) bay scallops, muscle removed

Mixed microgreens

2 ounces lemon oil

8 ounces Tomato Coulis (see below)

4–6 sprigs fresh thyme, leaves only

2 ounces red pear tomatoes

2 ounces yellow pear tomatoes

4 ounces Bruno Rossi tomatoes

4–6 sprigs thyme

3 ounces extra-virgin olive oil

Salt and pepper to taste

1. Cook lentils in water with bay leaf and garlic for 10–15 minutes. Strain lentils and set aside. Discard bay leaf and garlic.

2. Portion turkey bacon into 12 small slices, then sauté over medium heat until crispy. Set aside on paper towel to drain any excess oil.

3. Heat sauté pan with half of the butter and olive oil. Add chopped shallots, zucchini, yellow squash and green beans and sauté 3–5 minutes. Add cooked lentils, salt and pepper and sauté for another 3–5 minutes, then remove from heat and set aside.

4. Heat remaining olive oil and butter in sauté pan. Season scallops with salt and pepper, then sear scallops on high heat for less than a minute per side, until just carmelized. Save pan drippings and fold into lentil mixture.

5. Dress mixed microgreens with lemon oil and season with salt and pepper.

6. Place microgreens on one side of the plate. Streak the other side of the plate with tomato coulis and thyme sprigs. Place lentils on the middle of the plate, then place scallops on top of lentils. Garnish with turkey bacon.

TOMATO COULIS

Add all ingredients together in a blender and combine until smooth in consistency.

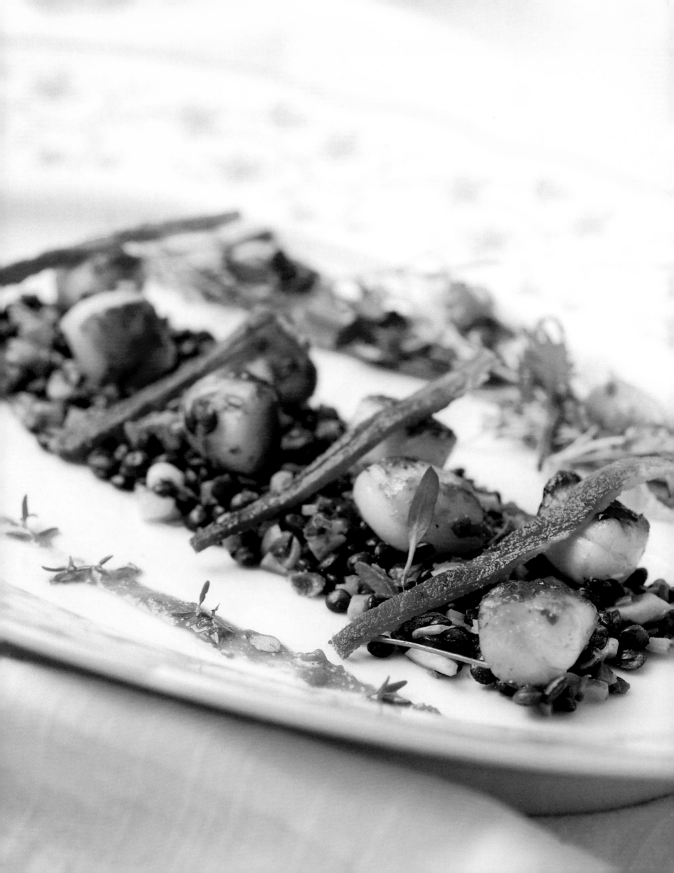

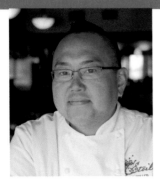

Tory Miller

Tory Miller is the executive chef & co-proprietor of L'Etoile Restaurant in Madison, Wisconsin, where his culinary creations begin with locally grown, sustainable and organic ingredients cultivated by numerous Wisconsin farmers. At L'Etoile, dinner menus always feature local ingredients, and a Wisconsin map hangs on the wall to show guests where their dinner comes from. Miller dedicates most of his free time to his partnership with Wisconsin Homegrown Lunch, advocating for fresh, local foods in the school system.

ROASTED WILD ALASKAN HALIBUT WITH GRILLED SWEET CORN SUCCOTASH

6 ears sweet corn

1 red onion

2 tablespoons extra-virgin olive oil

Salt and pepper

1 zucchini

1 red bell pepper

8 Sun Gold tomatoes

1 cup fresh edamame

1 tablespoon red wine vinegar

½ teaspoon chopped chives

½ teaspoon parsley

4 5-ounce fillets wild halibut

Canola oil

1. **Peel back the outer layers of the corn, but don't remove them completely. Remove the silk strands and fold back the husk. Soak the ears in cold water for about 20 minutes. Place on a hot grill for about 3 minutes on a side. (The outside will burn.) Set aside.**

2. **Peel and slice the onion into ¼-inch slices. Drizzle with about ½ tablespoon olive oil and season with salt and pepper. Grill the onion on high for about 2 minutes per side. Set aside.**

3. **Slice the zucchini into ¼-inch slices, season and cook like the onion.**

4. **Dice the red pepper into ⅛-inch squares. Slice the tomatoes in half.**

5. **Remove the corn from the cob into a large bowl.**

6. **Dice the zucchini and onions and add to the bowl.**

7. **Blanch the edamame to remove the pod, and then add to the bowl.**

8. **Stir in the reserved olive oil, vinegar and herbs. Add the peppers and tomatoes.**

9. **Preheat the oven to 475°F.**

10. **Heat a large, oven-safe pan over high heat. Season the halibut fillets with salt and pepper to taste. Add the canola oil to the hot pan and sear the fillets on the flesh side. Place the pan in oven for 6–7 minutes.**

11. **Plate the fish alongside the corn mixture.**

Yield: 4 servings

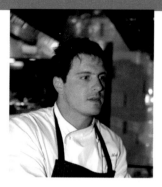

Seamus Mullen

Yearning to re-create the casual bars and *cervecerías* that Mullen discovered while living in Spain, he opened Boqueria, an accessible Spanish tapas restaurant in New York City, in August 2006. Based on the success of the original Flatiron District location, Mullen opened Boqueria SoHo in fall 2008. Seamlessly integrating local ingredients and house-cured meats with classic Spanish techniques and flavors, Boqueria's regional Spanish cuisine has been praised by both critics and patrons alike, earning a glowing two-star review from the *New York Times*.

PULPO MARINERO (OCTOPUS, RAZOR CLAMS, LA RATTE POTATOES AND SMOKED TOMATO BROTH)

8 littleneck clams

1 cup Manzanilla sherry

4 beefsteak tomatoes, lightly smoked in a hot smoker, then pureed

4 cups shellfish stock

8 razor clams

1 cup La Ratte potatoes, blanched and peeled

Salt

Pepper

Sherry vinegar

8 large octopus tentacles, tenderized and blanched

4 breakfast radishes, sliced on a mandolin

1 bunch oregano

1. **Place the littleneck clams and sherry in a large pot and steam uncovered for 3 minutes.**

2. **Add the pureed smoked tomatoes, shellfish stock, razor clams and potatoes and cover. Steam for 3 minutes until all the shellfish have opened. Check the broth for seasoning and adjust with salt, pepper and sherry vinegar.**

3. **While the shellfish are cooking, heat a grill or grill pan and cook the octopus tentacles, seasoned with salt and pepper, until golden and crispy.**

4. **In a deep bowl, spoon a small amount of the broth, a quarter of the potatoes, and two each of razor clams and littlenecks. Finish with two octopus tentacles and garnish with sliced radishes and oregano leaves.**

Yield: 4 servings

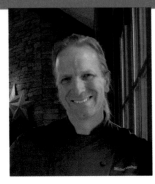

Michel Nischan

Michel Nischan is an advocate for a more healthful, organic and sustainable food future. A two-time James Beard Foundation award winner, Nischan is chef and owner of Dressing Room: A Homegrown Restaurant, located in Westport, Connecticut, and also president and CEO of Wholesome Wave Foundation, a nonprofit organization focused on making locally and sustainably grown foods available to all.

CURED SALMON WITH CARAMELIZED CAULIFLOWER

1 tablespoon coriander seeds, toasted

1 dried cascabel, Anaheim or New Mexico chili

1 tablespoon Sichuan peppercorns

½ cup raw cane sugar

¼ cup coarse sea salt or kosher salt

½ teaspoon freshly ground pepper

1¾ pounds skinless, boneless salmon fillet

From *Taste, Pure and Simple* (Chronicle Books, 2003)

CURED SALMON

1. Preheat the oven to 350°F.

2. In a small dry skillet, toast the coriander seeds over medium heat, shaking the pan, until they are lightly browned and aromatic, 2 to 3 minutes. Transfer to a plate and let cool.

3. Roast the chili in the oven for 10 to 15 minutes, or until aromatic. Let cool completely. Tear up the chili and put the pieces in a spice grinder. Add the toasted coriander seeds and Sichuan peppercorns and grind them all together until fine. Some pepper flakes will not break down, which is okay.

4. In a small bowl, combine the raw sugar, salt and pepper. Add the ground spice mixture and stir until blended. You should have 1 scant cup of cure. Cut a piece of parchment or waxed paper large enough to cover a baking sheet. Sprinkle half the cure over the center of the paper in roughly the shape of the salmon fillet. Put the fish on top and cover it with the remaining cure. Wrap securely in the paper and refrigerate for 2 to 2½ hours.

Yield: 4 servings

⅓ cup tahini, room temperature

2 tablespoons fresh lemon juice

1 garlic clove, crushed

1 teaspoon grated lemon zest

1 teaspoon grated lime zest

¼ teaspoon salt

Dash of cayenne pepper

¼ cup very hot water

1 2¾- to 3-pound cauliflower

2½ tablespoons grapeseed oil

Coarse salt

Freshly ground pepper

Lemon and lime wedges

Chervil or parsley sprigs

TAHINI SAUCE

5. Put the tahini in a blender or food processor and add the lemon juice, garlic, lemon and lime zests, salt and cayenne and blend well. With the machine running, add the water. Transfer to a bowl and let stand for 30 to 60 minutes to allow the flavor to develop.

CARAMELIZED CAULIFLOWER

6. Remove the green leaves and stem from the cauliflower. Cut off enough of the central core so the vegetable can stand upright. Cut down through the center of the cauliflower to divide the center into 4 slices, each ¾ to 1 inch thick. Reserve the florets from either side for another use. Gather up all the tiny bits of cauliflower on the cutting board and reserve them.

7. In a large cast-iron skillet, heat 1 tablespoon of the grapeseed oil over medium-high heat. Add the cauliflower slices in a single layer. Season lightly with salt and pepper. Place another heavy skillet on top of the slices to weigh them down, and press gently. Cook for about 5 minutes, rotating the skillet and pressing down occasionally, until the cauliflower slices are deeply browned on the bottom.

8. Add the reserved cauliflower bits and drizzle the remaining 1½ tablespoons grapeseed oil over the uncooked side of the cauliflower slices. Turn and cook for 4 to 5 minutes to brown on the second side. Reduce the heat slightly if the cauliflower seems to be browning too fast.

9. Light a fire in a charcoal grill, preheat a gas grill to medium hot or preheat the boiler. Scrape most of the cure off the fish, leaving a little for flavor. Cut the fish into 4 equal squares. Grill (skin side up) or broil (skin side down) for 2 to 3 minutes on each side, or until lightly browned on the outside and just slightly translucent in the center. Squeeze about 1 tablespoon each of lemon and lime juice over each piece of salmon.

10. Put a square of cauliflower in the center of each of 4 dinner plates. Arrange the salmon on top. Drizzle the tahini sauce around the fish and garnish with chervil or parsley.

SWEET POTATO AND ROOT VEGETABLE GRATIN

1 tablespoon extra-virgin olive oil

1 large rutabaga (about 1 pound), peeled and thinly sliced

1 pound russet potatoes, peeled

1½ pounds sweet potatoes, peeled and thinly sliced

1 cup shredded Vidalia onions

1 pound large parsnips, peeled and thinly sliced

1 tablespoon minced fresh herbs, such as flat-leaf parsley, thyme, chives and/or chervil

Salt

Freshly ground pepper

1 cup Sweet Potato Sauce (see below)

3½ cups sweet potato juice (approx. 1¼ pounds sweet potatoes will yield 1 cup of juice)

2 tablespoons fresh ginger

1 Thai chili, seeded and minced

Fresh lemon juice

Coarse salt

Freshly ground pepper

From *Taste, Pure and Simple* (Chronicle Books, 2003)

1. Preheat oven to 350°F. Rub an 8½-by-12 inch casserole dish with olive oil.

2. Overlap half the rutabaga slices on the bottom of the casserole, making sure the slices do not overlap by more than ½ inch. Sprinkle lightly with salt and pepper.

3. Thinly slice 1 of the russet potatoes lengthwise and shingle the slices over the rutabaga. Season lightly with salt and pepper. Slice the potatoes as you use them to prevent them from discoloring and so that they retain their starch and nutrients.

4. Overlap the sweet potato slices over the russet potato. Season with salt and pepper.

5. Spread about 1/3 cup of the onions over the sweet potato slices, then overlap the parsnips over these.

6. Repeat the process, ending with sweet potato slices. Spray lightly with a little vegetable oil cooking spray, season with salt and pepper, cover tightly with aluminum foil, and bake for 40 to 50 minutes.

7. Remove the casserole from the oven and uncover. Spray lightly with a little more oil. Sprinkle with the minced herbs. Return, uncovered, to the oven for 15 to 20 minutes, or until the top layer is nicely browned. Remove from the oven. Let set for 10 to 15 minutes before slicing and serving.

8. Heat the sweet potato sauce gently and serve the gratin with a little sauce drizzled over each serving.

Yield: 6 servings

SWEET POTATO SAUCE

9. Juice the sweet potatoes and let juice stand for at least 4 hours at room temperature. This will allow much of the potato starch in the juice to settle.

10. Pour the juice through a fine-mesh sieve into a wide, shallow pan, being careful to leave the settled starch behind. Place the juice over medium heat and bring to a gentle boil. Reduce the heat and simmer 25 to 30 minutes, or until reduced to about 1 cup. During the first 5 to 10 minutes of cooking, additional potato starch will rise to the surface. Skim it off and discard. If using a relatively deep pan, this reduction could take up to 1 hour.

11. Remove from heat and stir in the ginger and chili. Stir until the sauce tastes spicy enough, then strain immediately through a fine-mesh sieve. Season with lemon juice, salt and pepper.

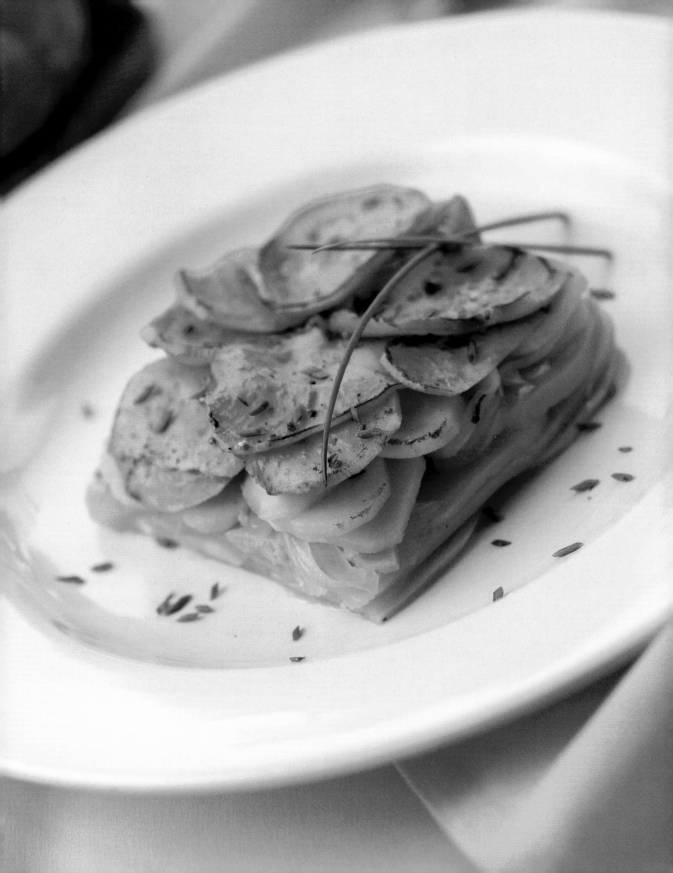

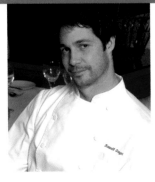

Ken Oringer

Ken Oringer is an award-winning chef and recipient of the 2001 James Beard American Express "Best Chef in the Northeast award." In 2002, Oringer added his acclaimed sashimi bar, Uni, to the lounge of his popular Boston restaurant, Clio. In 2005, both Clio and Uni were included in *Boston* magazine's list of the top twenty-five restaurants in the city. Since then, Oringer has opened Toro, a Barcelona-inspired tapas restaurant, and KO Prime, a modern steakhouse.

STEAMED BLACK BASS AND TOFU WITH HOT GARLIC OIL AND CHINESE BLACK BEANS

4 black bass fillets

8 ounces tofu, cut into 4 sheets

Black pepper

1 tablespoon lemon zest

1 tablespoon orange zest

3 tablespoons kaffir lime leaves, shredded

2 tablespoons Chinese black beans, chopped

¼ cup garlic oil (canola oil mixed with crushed garlic cloves to taste)

1 red jalapeño, stemmed and minced

1 serrano chile

3 ounces rice vinegar

1 bunch scallions, chopped

2 tablespoons soy sauce

2 bunches cilantro, chopped

2 tablespoons Korean pepper threads

1. **Preheat oven to 400°F.**

2. **Set up a bamboo steamer to accommodate all 4 fillets of black sea bass and a second layer to accommodate the tofu.**

3. **Season fillets on a plate with pepper. Scatter citrus zest, lime leaves and black beans on top of fish, then set aside.**

4. **When ready to steam, put the tofu slices on the bottom level of steamer and put fish fillets above, skin side up. Place steamer in bottom of oven and let steam until just cooked, about 8 minutes. When fish is done, place on serving tray.**

5. **While the fish is steaming, heat garlic oil until boiling.**

6. **When the fish has finished steaming, mix the cooking juices from the steamer with the jalapeño, serrano chile, rice wine vinegar, scallion, soy sauce and cilantro.**

7. **To serve, place tofu on plate, top with fish fillet, cover with sauce made from steaming juices and top with the hot garlic oil and Korean pepper threads.**

Yield: 4 servings

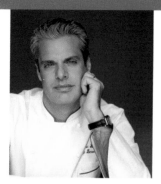

Eric Ripert

Eric Ripert was named "Outstanding Chef in the United States" by the James Beard Foundation in 2003. He is co-owner and executive chef of Le Bernardin, a four-star restaurant in New York City, as well as the Westend Bistro in Washington, D.C. He is also culinary director of and a partner in 10 ARTS in Philadelphia, as well as the author of the books *A Return to Cooking* and *On the Line*.

KANPACHI TARTARE TOPPED WITH WASABI TOBIKO, GINGER-CORIANDER EMULSION

2 teaspoons wasabi paste

1 tablespoon fresh lemon juice

3 tablespoons fresh lime juice

1½ tablespoons ginger oil

4 tablespoons canola oil

1 teaspoon sugar

Fine sea salt

Freshly ground white pepper

8 ounces kanpachi, ¼-inch dice

2 teaspoons wasabi paste

1 teaspoon ginger oil

1 teaspoon canola oil

1 teaspoon fresh lime juice

1 teaspoon fresh lemon juice

4 teaspoons fresh cilantro, julienne

Fine sea salt

Freshly ground white pepper

1 ounce wasabi tobiko

8 micro cilantro sprouts

GINGER-CORIANDER EMULSION

1. **Combine the wasabi, lemon juice and lime juice in a blender and process. Slowly emulsify in the ginger oil and the canola oil. Add the sugar and season to taste with salt and pepper. Reserve.**

KANPACHI TARTARE

2. **Combine the kanpachi, wasabi paste, ginger oil, canola oil, lime juice, lemon juice, cilantro, salt and pepper. Gently mix everything together and adjust the seasoning with salt and pepper. Gently fold 2 teaspoons of the wasabi tobiko into the tartare.**

3. **Mold ¼ cup of the kanpachi tartare into a 3-inch ring mold. Spread 1 teaspoon of wasabi tobiko on top of each tartare. Transfer the tartare to appetizer plates and remove the molds. Repeat until all the mixture has been used.**

4. **Garnish the top of each tartare with two micro cilantro sprouts. Spoon sauce around the tartare and serve immediately.**

Yield: 4 servings

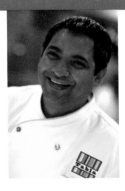

Floyd Cardoz

Floyd Cardoz is widely credited with putting Indian cuisine on the culinary map in New York City. After working at Lespinasse, Cardoz went on to open Tabla in 1998, where he is the executive chef and partner. In October 2006, Cardoz released his first cookbook, *One Spice, Two Spice*, and in January 2007, he received the first-ever "Humanitarian of the Year" award from Food TV and Share Our Strength in honor of his continued commitment to community engagement.

BENGALI FISH CURRY WITH EGGPLANT, POTATOES AND OKRA

1½ tablespoons coriander seeds, ground fine

1 teaspoon cumin seeds, ground fine

1 teaspoon brown mustard seeds, ground fine, or 1 teaspoon Coleman's mustard powder

1 teaspoon turmeric

¼ teaspoon cayenne

3 tablespoons canola oil

3 cloves

2 bay leaves

1 teaspoon whole brown mustard seeds

3 cups quartered and thinly sliced white onion

2 tablespoons minced peeled ginger

1 tablespoon minced garlic

4 large vine-ripe beefsteak tomatoes, seeded and chopped (about 4 cups)

Sea salt

2 fresh green chiles (seranos), slit down 1 side

½ cup dry white wine

1½ quarts fish stock, vegetable stock or water

1 large Japanese eggplant (about 6 ounces), cut into large bite-sized pieces (about 2 cups)

1 cup carrots cut into ½-inch dice

2 large Yukon Gold potatoes, cut into large bite-sized pieces (about 2 cups)

½ pound okra, trimmed

6 6-ounce pieces wild striped bass or cod fillet with skin

Freshly ground black pepper

1 cup cilantro leaves, cut into ribbons

1. Combine the spices in a small bowl and stir in 2 tablespoons water to make a paste.

2. Heat the oil in a 5–6-quart pan over moderately high heat until it simmers and add the cloves, bay leaves and whole mustard seeds. Cook, stirring, until the mustard seeds pop and the spices are fragrant, about 30 seconds. Stir in the onion, ginger and garlic and cook until the onion is translucent, about 5 minutes. Add the spice paste, tomatoes and 2½ teaspoons salt and cook, stirring, until the tomatoes are softened, about 2 minutes. Add the green chile, white wine and fish stock and bring the sauce to a boil. The curry can be made up to this point 1 day ahead, cooled completely, uncovered, and refrigerated, covered.

3. Bring the sauce to a boil and add the eggplant, carrots, potatoes and okra. Simmer the sauce until the vegetables are tender, about 20 minutes.

4. Season the fish with salt and pepper and let sit for 5 minutes. Completely submerge the fish in the sauce and bring to a boil. Simmer the curry for 5 minutes, then turn off the heat and tightly cover the pan. Let sit for 5 minutes longer. Sprinkle with the cilantro.

Yield: 6 servings

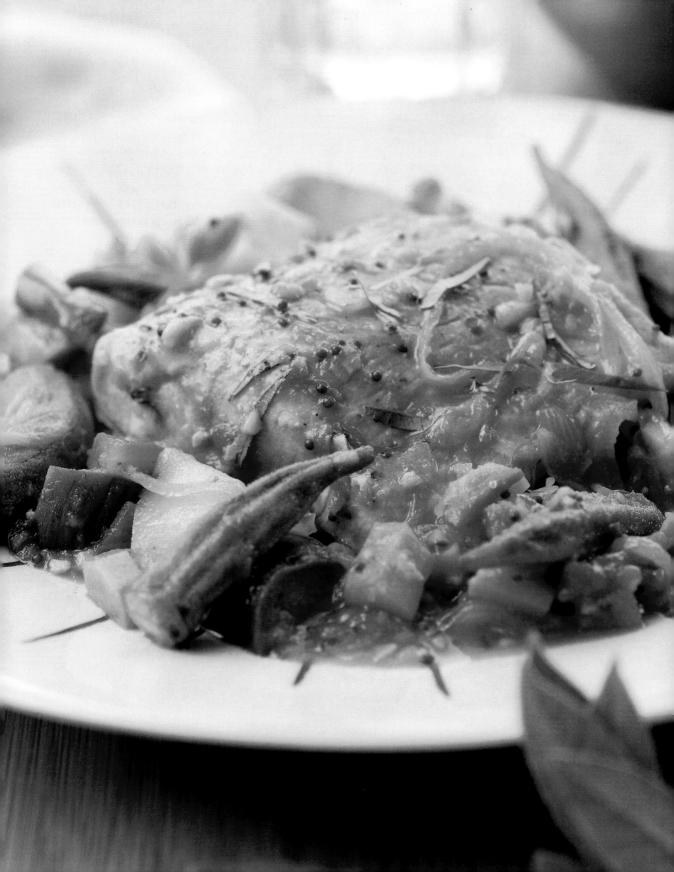

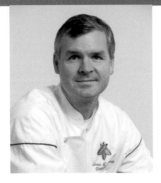

Andrew G. Shotts

Andrew G. Shotts, of Garrison Confections in Providence, Rhode Island, is one of the nation's premier chocolatiers. He blends innovation with years of talent honed at restaurants such as the Russian Tea Room and La Côte Basque in New York City. Garrison Confections has garnered national attention on the Food Network and in publications such as *Food & Wine* and *USA TODAY*.

APPLE AND PEACH CRUMBLE

FILLING

3 cups cubed Granny Smith apples

3 cups cubed fresh peaches

½ cup Splenda

2 tablespoons cornstarch

¼ teaspoon cinnamon

¼ teaspoon nutmeg

¼ teaspoon ginger

Juice of one orange

Zest of one orange

TOPPING

1½ cups uncooked old-fashioned oats

⅔ cup Splenda

4 tablespoons melted butter

½ teaspoon cinnamon

Pinch salt

1. Preheat oven to 375°F.

2. Combine all of the ingredients for the filling together and toss well, then pour into a 9-inch pie dish.

3. Bake for 20 minutes until fruit is soft.

4. Mix all of the ingredients for the topping together well.

5. Remove dish from oven and cover with the topping.

6. Bake again for another 10 to 15 minutes until top is crisp and lightly brown.

7. Let cool for 15 minutes before serving.

Yield: 8 servings

INTERVIEW WITH SAM TALBOT, A DIABETIC CHEF

Dr. S: When were you first diagnosed with diabetes?

Sam: Twelve years old.

Dr. S: What foods were you told you had to give up because of the diabetes?

Sam: The obvious ones—the cakes, the candies and all that kind of jazz. The things that kind of came as a shock were the mashed potatoes, the french fries. You know kids love mashed potatoes and french fries.

Dr. S: What foods do you miss the most because of your diabetes?

Sam: I really don't miss any of them. Occasionally, I will have something that I shouldn't, but life's a balancing act.

Dr. S: What's your favorite comfort food as a diabetic?

Sam: That's a good question. I have to really be honest—I love french fries.

Dr. S: What was your favorite comfort food when you were a kid?

Sam: Chicken fingers.

Dr. S: What was your least favorite food when you were a kid?

Sam: Brussels sprouts.

Dr. S: As a diabetic, which six foods would you want if you were stranded on a desert island?

Sam: Onions, garlic, broccoli, striped bass, apples and bananas.

Dr. S: What's the most unusual combination of foods that you eat?

Sam: Blueberries, crab and popcorn.

Dr. S: What advice would you have for a child with diabetes?

Sam: Always monitor your blood sugar. It's just an extra chore like washing your face—it only takes a couple of seconds.

Dr. S: What's your favorite smell in the kitchen?

Sam: Roasted garlic.

Dr. S: What's your favorite seasoning?

Sam: Sea salt.

Dr. S: When did you decide you wanted to be a chef?

Sam: When I was sixteen.

Dr. S: Do you cook at home?

Sam: I do—I cook a lot of vegetarian foods.

Dr. S: What unusual situation has happened to you surrounding food?

Sam: I was about twenty years old, cooking in a restaurant, and my mentor came into the kitchen where we were cooking. We had been cooking all night. I put a dish in the window that looked like a pork chop. My mentor—the executive chef—looked at the pork chop and called my name. I said, "Yes, Chef. Yes, Chef," and he said, "Sam, would you serve that to your mother?" and I kind of looked around to see if there was something I should notice and said, "Yes, Chef." He said, "Would you serve that to my mother? Would you serve that to my mother?" I looked at him—I didn't think there was anything wrong with it and I said, "Yes, Chef." Then he said, twice, "Are you sure about that?" I said, "Yes, Chef, I am. I think it looks great." He said, "Good—because your mother and my mother are sitting at the table and I wanted to make sure!" I looked out and saw them sitting at the table and they were actually sitting together. I freaked out and the whole kitchen line died laughing.

Dr. S: Of anyone in the world you would most like to have dinner with—living or dead—who would it be? And why?

Sam: My grandfather. Because he's the man. When I was seventeen, I was just getting started and I was buying cookbooks and I was working at Dean and Deluca. Now I think as the years have progressed and this is my career, it would be an honor to actually show him what it is that I do.

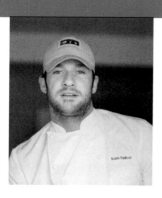

Sam Talbot

Sam Talbot began his career as the executive chef of the Black Duck Restaurant in New York City before he opened the Williamsburgh Cafe as chef and owner in Brooklyn, New York. In the summer of 2008, Talbot became the executive chef for the restaurant at The Surf Lodge in Montauk, New York, and created a menu of locally sourced, market-driven seafood. The restaurant is currently the most buzzed-about culinary destination on the east end of Long Island.

PICKLED WATERMELON SALAD WITH CHIMICHURRI VINAIGRETTE AND RICOTTA SALATA

3 cups water

2 cups watermelon pieces (cut from rind, seeded and cut into 1-inch cubes)

1 cup white vinegar

1 tablespoon honey or 1 packet Splenda

2 cinnamon sticks

¼ teaspoon ground ginger

1 tablespoon lemon juice

1 cup chopped fresh Italian parsley

½ cup olive oil

⅓ cup red wine vinegar

¼ cup basil, chopped

2 garlic cloves, peeled and mashed

¾ teaspoon crushed red pepper

1 teaspoon lemon zest

1 teaspoon lime zest

Salt and pepper to taste

4 ounces ricotta salata

MELON

1. Mix all of the ingredients in a large bowl.

2. Add the watermelon and let stand overnight.

3. Drain the watermelon, rinse and drain again.

4. In a large saucepan, combine the vinegar, sugar, cinnamon stick, ginger and lemon juice. Bring to a boil and simmer for 20 minutes. Then add watermelon to warm liquid and let it sit until room temperature. Place in container and refrigerate.

Makes 4 servings

VINAIGRETTE

5. Mix all ingredients except the ricotta salata in a large mixing bowl and whisk until incorporated.

6. Arrange the melon on a plate. Spoon the vinaigrette over the top.

7. Take a cheese grater and skim the ricotta over the fine side a few times for the final garnish.

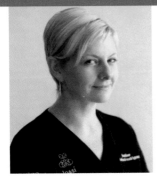

Heather Carlucci-Rodriguez

Celebrated for her three-star desserts, Heather Carlucci-Rodriguez's pastry-chef résumé reads like a history of New York's most esteemed eateries. She has created desserts at L'Impero, Veritas and Judson Grill, each receiving three stars from the *New York Times*. For her first personal venture, Heather opened Lassi, a tiny takeout restaurant featuring Northern Indian home cooking. In March 2006 *New York* magazine named Lassi "Best Take-Out" in New York City.

CHANA DAL

1 cup chana or mung dal

4 cups water

13 chiles, finely chopped

¼ teaspoon turmeric

1 teaspoon salt

1 teaspoon cumin seeds

1 tablespoon canola oil

1½ onions, finely chopped

1 tablespoon ginger, chopped

1½ teaspoons salt

1 tablespoon coriander, ground

½ teaspoon ground cumin

¼ teaspoon paprika

2 tablespoons chopped cilantro

1. **Combine dal, water, chiles, turmeric and 1 teaspoon salt and bring to a boil. Add more water if needed as dal cooks until soft.**

2. **Cook cumin seeds in oil to sizzle. Caramelize onions with cumin. Add ginger and cook until soft.**

3. **Add 1½ teaspoons salt, coriander, ground cumin and paprika and cook through. Pour over dal and stir.**

4. **Finish with cilantro.**

Yield: 4 servings

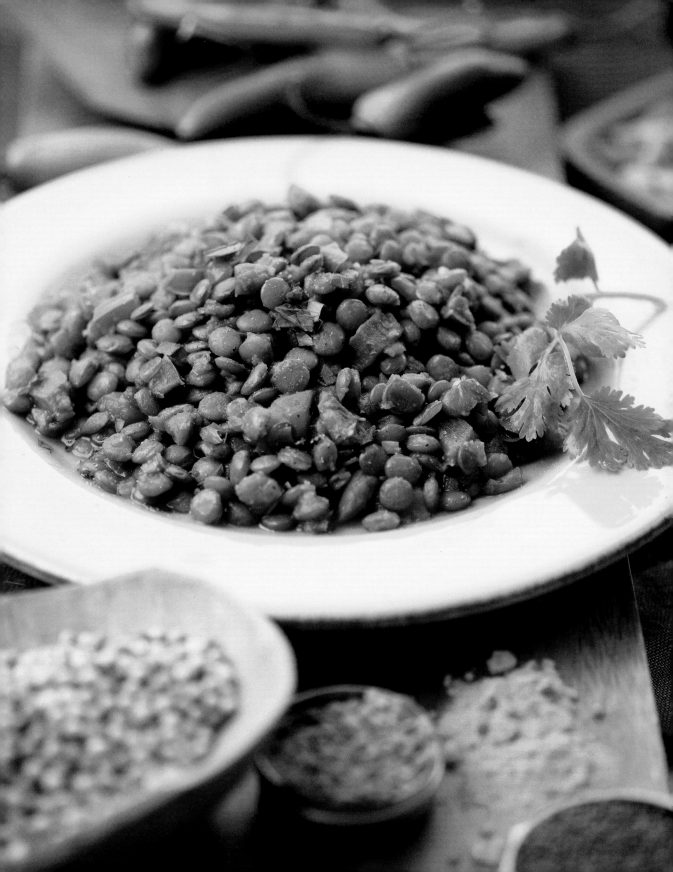

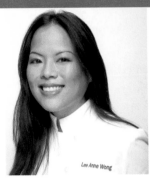

Lee Anne Wong

After graduating from the French Culinary Institute and immersing herself in the restaurant world, Lee Anne Wong returned to the FCI as the executive chef of event operations. Wong brought her culinary skills to an even wider audience when she appeared as a contestant on Season One of Bravo's *Top Chef*. The show's producers saw her innate talent and media experience and brought her on as the show's supervising culinary producer.

STEAMED BASS, RADISH SALAD, SHISO AND PONZU

4 5-ounce pieces boneless skinless bass fillet

1 tablespoon yuzu juice

2 tablespoons vegetable oil

Salt

White pepper

Banana leaf for wrapping

8 pieces shiso leaf

4 scallions, white and greens, julienned into 2-inch matchsticks

1 piece ginger, peeled, julienned into 2-inch matchsticks

STEAMED FISH

1. Pat the fish fillets dry. In a small bowl, whisk together the yuzu juice and oil. Brush both sides of each fillet with the vinaigrette. Season lightly with salt and pepper.

2. Cut pieces of banana leaf large enough to wrap each fillet completely. Place a piece of shiso on the banana leaf. Place the fish fillet on top of the shiso and top with another shiso leaf. Top the fillets with a generous pinch of scallion and ginger. Carefully wrap each fillet in the banana leaf to make a package and tie securely with butcher's twine.

3. Place the packets in a steamer basket approximately 3 inches over boiling water. Cover with a tight-fitting lid. Steam the fillets for 8 minutes, until just cooked through. Unwrap the fish and discard the aromatics. Serve immediately with Root Vegetable Salad and Ponzu Sauce.

Yield: 4 servings

1 red beet, peeled

1 daikon or watermelon radish, peeled

1 sweet potato, peeled

1 tablespoon olive oil

1 teaspoon yuzu juice

¼ teaspoon sugar

1 tablespoon shiso leaf, fine chiffonade

Salt

Black pepper

1 cup sudachi juice (or a mixture of lemon and lime)

⅓ cup plus 2 tablespoons rice vinegar

1 cup plus 2 tablespoons soy sauce

3 tablespoons mirin

1 tablespoon dried bonito flakes

1 piece konbu, cut into a 2-inch square

ROOT VEGETABLE SALAD

4. Julienne all of the vegetables to ⅛-inch thick matchsticks, about 3 inches in length.

5. Combine the olive oil, yuzu juice and sugar in a bowl, whisking until the sugar dissolves.

6. Toss the vegetables and shiso leaf in the vinaigrette. Season generously with salt and pepper. Serve immediately on top of the steamed fish fillet.

PONZU SAUCE

7. Mix all ingredients together and refrigerate for 24 hours. Strain the solids through a fine cheesecloth or chinois.

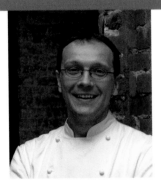

Bill Telepan

Bill Telepan graduated from the Culinary Institute of America. Inspired by his exceptional reviews and strong following as the executive chef at Gotham Bar & Grill in New York City, Telepan published the book *Inspired by Ingredients* to present his unique cooking style and most popular recipes. In December of 2005, Telepan opened his eponymous restaurant Telepan on the Upper West Side of Manhattan, which was voted Best Newcomer by the Zagat Survey in 2007.

ZUCCHINI AND TOMATO EGG WHITE FRITTATA WITH WILD ARUGULA AND GOLD NUGGET POTATOES

3 tablespoons olive oil

½ pound Gold Nugget potatoes

4 sprigs thyme, plus 2 teaspoons chopped fresh thyme for frittata

½ Walla Walla onion, finely chopped

2 garlic cloves

1 tomato, peeled, seeded and chopped

Whites of 12 eggs

1 medium zucchini, halved and thinly sliced

1 ounce arugula

Salt

1. Place 1 tablespoon oil, potatoes, sprigs of thyme and a good pinch of salt onto a large piece of foil, fold up and place on top of a grill or under a broiler and cook until potatoes are tender, about 12–15 minutes. Reserve.

2. Heat 1 tablespoon oil in a 10-inch sauté pan over medium heat. Add onion and garlic and a pinch of salt and soften for about 5–7 minutes.

3. Add tomato and cook until all moisture is removed, about 8–10 minutes. Add zucchini and chopped thyme, mix together and cook an additional 3 minutes. Take off the heat, place in bowl and allow to cool to room temperature.

4. Whisk the egg whites. Mix in the zucchini.

5. Heat remaining oil in a 10-inch sauté pan on medium heat, add the egg-zucchini mixture and cook until edges start to solidify. Place in oven until the frittata is cooked through, about 12–15 minutes.

6. Slip onto cutting board, cut into serving wedges (4–8), place on top of arugula and serve with the potatoes.

Yield: 4 servings

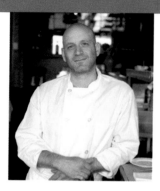

Marc Vetri

Marc Vetri was named one of *Food & Wine*'s ten best new chefs in 2005 and received the *Philadelphia Inquirer*'s highest restaurant rating. In 2005, Vetri won the James Beard Award for "Best Chef Mid-Atlantic." He is the chef and owner of Vetri and Osteria, two popular restaurants in Philadelphia. The story of Vetri's culinary journey, along with the recipes for his most popular dishes, have been collected in his book, *Il Viaggio Di Vetri: A Culinary Journey.*

FUSILLI PASTA SALAD WITH JUMBO CRAB

2 ounces jumbo lump crab meat

½ cup fusilli, cooked al dente (preferably whole grain)

¼ cup pear tomatoes, halved

¼ cup celery, thinly sliced

2 tablespoons light mayonnaise

2 tablespoons tarragon

1 teaspoon lemon juice

Salt

Pepper

¼ cup mâche or bibb lettuce

1. Combine crab, pasta, tomatoes, celery, mayonnaise, tarragon, lemon, salt and pepper in bowl.

2. Place mâche evenly across plate.

3. Place salad mixture over mâche.

4. Place tarragon over top of salad.

5. Finish with fresh cracked pepper.

Yield: 1 serving

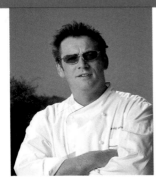

David Walzog

David Walzog is a three-time nominee for the James Beard/Perrier-Jouet Rising Chef Award. He was the corporate executive chef for the Glazier Group in New York City and was at the helm of New York's legendary Steakhouse at Monkey Bar, as well as the Michael Jordan Steakhouse and three Strip House restaurants. Under his supervision, *New York* magazine claimed Strip House to have the "Best Steak in New York" in 2001, and *Forbes* magazine named the restaurant one of "Forbes 2003 All-Star Eateries in New York." Walzog is currently the executive chef of SW Steakhouse in Las Vegas.

STEAMED PRAWNS WITH LEMON, SEAWEED AND AROMATIC VEGETABLES

4 ounces seaweed, rinsed

12 red prawns, head on, peeled of the tail shell

8 ounces light beer

1 tablespoon celery seed

2 teaspoons paprika

1 red bell pepper, seeded and julienned

1 white onion, cut in half and thinly sliced

1 carrot, peeled and thinly sliced

1 lemon, thinly sliced

1. Use a stove-top-safe deep casserole dish with a lid. Add the seaweed to the bottom of the dish to create a raft for the prawns to steam on top of. Add the prawns on top of the seaweed and then add the remaining ingredients in the order listed at left.

2. Place the dish over medium-high heat on the stove-top and allow to steam for 8 minutes.

3. Remove from heat and let stand with the lid closed for an additional 2–3 minutes before serving.

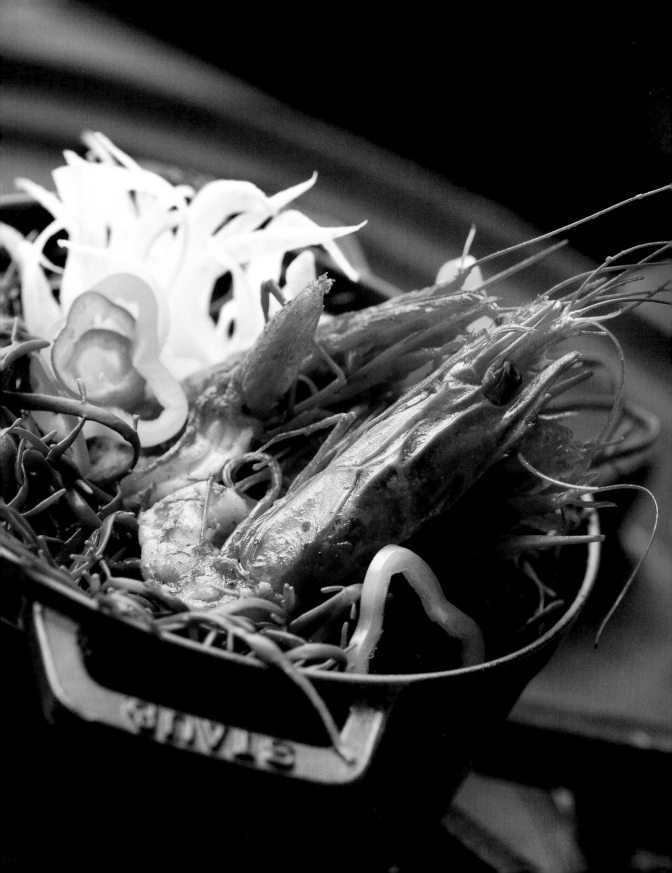

CHAPTER 11

Beating Diabetes Every Day

You now know how to beat diabetes. You've seen—literally—the choices that can help you prevent or manage the disease, choices that can cancel out the damaging, sometimes fatal impact of diabetes. All you have to do now is go out and make the right choices.

We have a few things to say that may help. For we know that despite all the information you've just absorbed, you probably have some questions about how to put the information to work on a daily basis. Questions like:

- What does "eating the Pyramid way" look like day after day?
- How can I make the right choices when I confront a restaurant menu? How about a fast-food restaurant menu?
- What about supplements?
- If I eat the Pyramid way, do I really need to exercise?

So here are a few more resources that can help you translate the science, the medical warnings and the food-specific information of the previous chapters into simple, practical advice for beating diabetes on a day-to-day basis.

EATING CHOICES

Eating is a matter of choosing. Seeing the difference between food options can help you make more healthful choices for a slimmer, stronger you. The chart below shows you some different eating options—and the difference your choice can make.

CALORIES

½ ounce reduced-fat cookies	= 70 =	1½ pounds watermelon
1 mouthful bacon cheeseburger (approx. one-fifth)	= 190 =	1 veggie burger on light bun with catsup, onion, relish
1-inch cube reduced-fat cheese	= 100 =	1 banana

1 ounce pâté	= 135 =	3 ounces smoked salmon
1 croissant	= 400 =	4 light English muffins
1 chocolate truffle	= 90 =	3 chocolate-dipped strawberries
1 cup orange juice	= 110 =	3 oranges
1 Tofutti Cutie	= 120 =	4 Tofutti Chocolate Fudge Treats
1 serving General Tso's chicken (10 ounce)	= 960 =	4 servings shrimp and Chinese vegetables in hoisin sauce
1 serving vegetable tempura	= 380 =	4 servings edamame
1 cup chicken salad	= 580 =	5 cups three-bean salad
1 egg roll	= 400 =	5 bowls hot-and-sour soup
1 tablespoon margarine	= 100 =	10 tablespoons sugar-free marmalade
1 ounce Swiss cheese	= 105 =	24 large olives

THE ALL-PYRAMID SEVEN-DAY MENU SAMPLE

What follows is not a diet. It is not a plan. No one is suggesting you follow it. Rather, it is a sample of what seven days of meals composed solely of foods from the Beat Diabetes Pyramid might look like. For every day, it offers a breakfast, lunch, snack and dinner menu.

This may not be the way you eat; perhaps, like one of the authors of this book, you tend not to eat breakfast. Or maybe, like the other author, you simply don't care for a sweet dessert after dinner.

Don't change your way of eating because of these meal plans. And of course, if you are diabetic, especially if you are on medication, before you make any changes in the way you eat, be sure to check with your doctor to see if you need to coordinate your food intake with your medication.

Mostly, however, *it's our hope that these twenty-eight menus*—seven different breakfasts, seven different lunches, seven different snacks and seven different dinners—*will give you the sense of the variety of menus that can be put together from the Beat Diabetes Pyramid.* They're a testament to the rich diversity of tastes and textures possible when you are fighting diabetes and strengthening your overall health.

SEVEN-DAY SAMPLE MENU

BREAKFAST	LUNCH	SNACK	DINNER

DAY 1

BREAKFAST	LUNCH	SNACK	DINNER
■ Cantaloupe ■ Veggie sausage patties on toasted light English muffin	■ Three-bean chili with onions, salsa and guacamole ■ Cucumber and tomato salad	■ Roasted soy nuts	■ Herb-grilled halibut ■ Green beans with almonds ■ Baked acorn squash ■ Fresh mango

DAY 2

BREAKFAST	LUNCH	SNACK	DINNER
■ Cinnamon baked apple ■ Oatmeal with chopped walnuts	■ Marukome miso soup with soba noodles ■ Edamame ■ Sashimi with wasabi and pickled ginger ■ Seaweed salad	■ Baby carrots with hummus dip	■ Whole-grain spaghetti and veggie meatballs with marinara sauce ■ Sautéed eggplant and zucchini ■ Sugar-free frozen fruit bars

DAY 3

BREAKFAST	LUNCH	SNACK	DINNER
■ Sliced orange ■ Smoked salmon on light toast with tomato	■ Black bean soup ■ Veggie burger on whole-grain roll with catsup and relish ■ Sliced tomatoes and onion	■ Pistachio nuts	■ Hot-and-sour soup ■ Shrimp and mixed Chinese vegetables in hoisin sauce ■ Fresh pineapple

DAY 4

BREAKFAST	LUNCH	SNACK	DINNER
■ Blueberries ■ Whole-grain waffles with pecans and sugar-free maple syrup	■ Green pea soup ■ Tuna salad on greens with tomatoes, cucumbers, etc.	■ Apple slices with peanut butter	■ Marinated artichoke hearts ■ Veggie Italian sausages and peppers ■ Broccoli rabe with garlic and olive oil ■ Sugar-free frozen fudge pops

SEVEN-DAY SAMPLE MENU

BREAKFAST	LUNCH	SNACK	DINNER
DAY 5			
• Mixed fruit cup • Spanish omelet with peppers, onions, olives and tomato sauce (preferably made with egg whites or egg substitute) • Light toast	• Butternut squash soup • Spinach salad with mushrooms, chickpeas, beets, avocado and toasted pumpkin seeds	• Edamame	• Manhattan clam chowder • Grilled salmon • Roasted cauliflower and asparagus • Lemon-Berry Parfait (see recipe on page 116)
DAY 6			
• Mauve Madness, a soy milk shake with blackberries and blueberries (see recipe on page 40)	• Mulligatawny soup (spiced lentil soup) • Chana saag (curried chickpeas and spinach) • Cucumber raita and chutney	• Toasted sunflower seeds	• Blackened tuna • Roasted beets • Corn on the cob • Poached pear
DAY 7			
• Whole-grain pancakes with sliced banana and peanut butter	• Baked potato with red bean chili and pico de gallo • Baby greens salad	• Mixed pepper slices with roasted eggplant dip	• Carrot-ginger soup • Sesame Tofu and Vegetable Stir-Fry (see recipe on page 198) • Strawberries and kiwi fruit

BEATING DIABETES WHILE DINING OUT

Dining out—whether at Chez Haute Cuisine, at the fast-food chain on the highway or at the deli on the way to work—doesn't mean giving up on the fight against diabetes and for weight loss. Take a look at these **partial** menus from a variety of our favorite restaurants around New York City—among the very best in New York City—and see how we've highlighted the choices that can keep you on the Pyramid. As they say about New York, if you can beat diabetes there, you can do it anywhere.

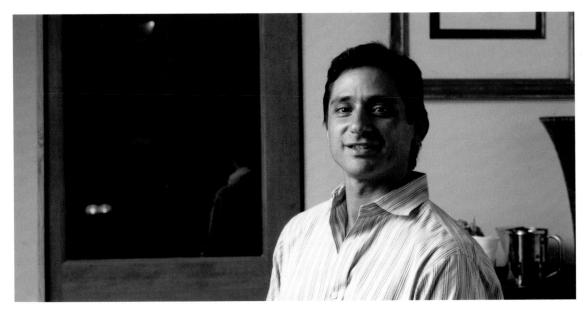

41 Greenwich

The vintage orange plaid wallpaper from the sixties gives dining at 41 Greenwich the feeling of coming home. The dining room is familiar and welcoming, much like the menu.

The owner, Jay Plumeri, built the business the old-fashioned way—one guest at a time, through word of mouth. New Yorkers keep returning to 41 Greenwich because they appreciate the food as much as the owners love to make it. Many friends have been made in this cozy space, which is a labor of love, providing creative and healthy cuisine.

MENU

STARTERS

Iceberg Wedge
Roquefort, scallion and bacon

Brussels Sprout Salad
With frisee, lemon, olive oil, red onion,
Roquefort and reggiano

Grilled Shrimp
Over avocado and jalapeño salsa

Crab Cake
Jumbo lump, mango and apple chutney

Prosciutto di Parma
Mission figs, goat cheese and olive oil

Roasted Beet & Pumpkin Salad
With arugula, radicchio, balsamic and
toasted pine nuts

Tuna Tartare
Sesame, radish, soy and scallion

Chopped Salad
Mesclun, provolone, red onion, tomato,
salami, cucumbers and black olives

Fish Taco
Daily fish, tomato, cilantro, lime, lemon,
red onion rolled in soft tortilla

MAINS

Beef Carpaccio
Arugula, lemon mustard and shaved reggiano

Joe's Chopped Lobster Salad
Romaine, hearts of palm, red onion, tomato
and avocado

Grilled Salmon
Citrus zest with dill and zucchini salad

Lemon Sole
Filet with caper, white wine and spinach

Chicken Jones
With house rub, haricot vert and garlic
mashed potatoes

Pork Chop
Double-cut with thyme, coriander and
cinnamon-stewed apples

***Sea Scallops Over Chopped Seasonal
Root Vegetables**

Lobster Tagliolini
Chopped tomato, shallots, basil and a touch
of cream

Macaroni & Cheese
Bacon or lobster

Filet Mignon (8 ounces)
With port mushroom sauce

Burgers (8 ounces)
Homemade potato chips

SIDES

Sautéed spinach

Mushrooms

Brussels sprouts

Couscous

Okra, tossed

Garlic mashed potato

Green beans, shallots and toasted pine nuts

Beat Diabetes approved items in orange.

*See recipe and photo for Sea Scallops on pages 252–253.

SEA SCALLOPS OVER CHOPPED SEASONAL ROOT VEGETABLES

Extra-virgin olive oil

6 jumbo sea scallops

Ground rock salt

Freshly ground pepper

1 teaspoon butter

Squeeze of lemon juice

1 tablespoon chopped parsley

1 turnip, cut into ½-inch cubes

1 parsnip, cut into ½-inch cubes

2 carrots, cut into ½-inch cubes

1 stalk celery, cut into ½-inch cubes

1 garlic clove, crushed

1 tablespoon chopped chives

1. Pre-heat oven to 325°F.

2. Heat olive oil in skillet. Add scallops and sauté until golden brown. Season with salt and pepper. Add butter and lemon juice and cook for approximately 8 minutes, or until scallops are medium/rare. Just before you take the pan off the heat, add the chopped parsley. Remove scallops from the pan and set them on paper towels to drain excess oil.

3. In the same pan with the cooking juices, add vegetables and garlic. Sauté for a few minutes, then cover and cook until tender, approximately 10 minutes.

4. Return the scallops to the skillet with the vegetables and brown in oven for 5 minutes until scallops are almost cooked through.

5. Divide the dish onto 2 plates. Sprinkle with chives and a light drizzle of olive oil.

Yield: 2 servings

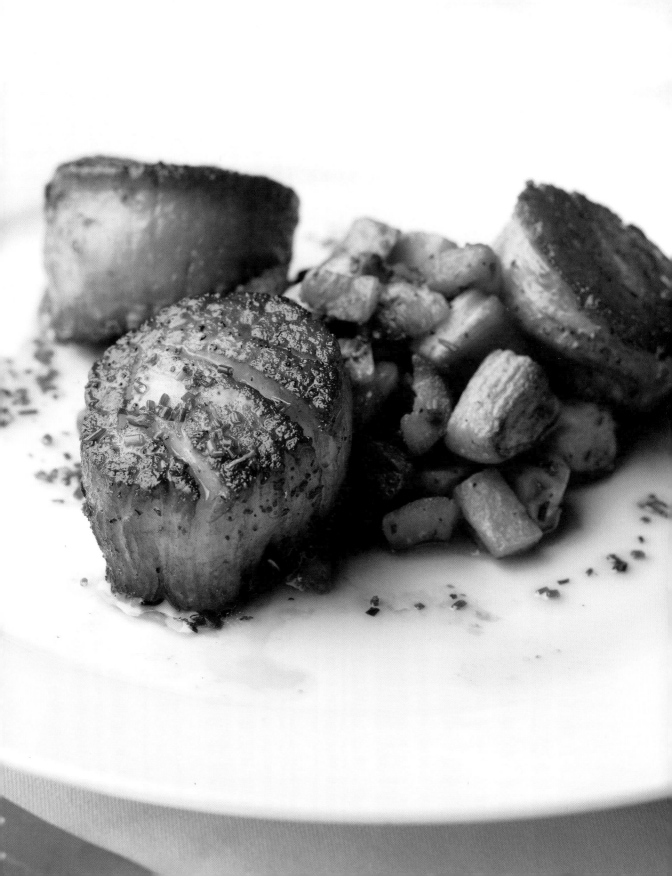

Le Cirque

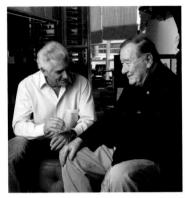

Dr. Shapiro consulting with Sirio Maccioni.

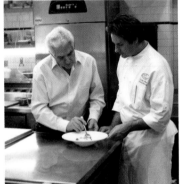

Dr. Shapiro tasting one of the menu items with Chef Craig Hopson at Le Cirque.

Sirio Maccioni is perhaps Manhattan's most charismatic restaurateur—the brains, the energy and the passion behind the legendary Le Cirque. Sirio Maccioni has dedicated his life to the restaurant business, and few have achieved the love and respect around the world that Le Cirque's ringmaster has.

Le Cirque was the first privately owned hotel restaurant in New York City. Maccioni presented to New York what quickly became its most favored restaurant, one frequented by politicians, entertainers, the social set, artists and royalty. Neither Maccioni nor his family have had time to look back since.

Sirio Maccioni continues to work each day and tends also to its sister restaurant, Osteria del Circo, also located in New York City. Le Cirque and Osteria del Circo are also located in Las Vegas at the Bellagio hotel, and a Beach Club by Le Cirque is part of Casa de Campo Resort in the Dominican Republic.

MENU

APPETIZERS

Le Cirque Salad

Marinated Tuna
Avocado tapenade, clementines and sesame tuile

Sautéed Gulf Shrimp
Forbidden rice, green papaya and curry yogurt sauce

Local Corn and Basil Soup
Crab-ricotta dumplings

Smoked Ham Hock and Parmesan Consommé
Prosciutto, fondue and conchilie

Wild Burgundy Escargot
Gruyère gnocchi, pickled chanterelles and bottarga

Torchon of Foie Gras
Strawberries, balsamic vinegar and crisp prosciutto

MENU

MAINS

Paupiette of Black Cod
Leeks, potatoes, Rocca di Frassinello sauce

*Halibut Poached in Coconut Milk
Mussels, chanterelles and saffron

Dover Sole
Meunière, almondine or grilled

Diver Sea Scallops
Foie gras sabayon, turnips and diable sauce

Warm Maine Lobster
Braised lobster mushrooms, hazelnut milk and curry

Chicken Breast
Corn, wood ear mushrooms and basil

Rack of Lamb
Black Mission figs and goat cheese panisse

Prime Dry-Aged Strip Steak
Bone marrow flan, sweet onion and lamb's quarters

TABLESIDE FOR TWO

Whole Roasted Turbot

Whole Roasted Chicken

SEAFOOD & CAVIAR

Plateau Fruits de Mer

Trio de Luxe

Half-Shell Oysters

Wild Golden Osetra Caviar
1 ounce

Californian Osetra Caviar
1 ounce

Scrambled Eggs with Caviar

CHEF'S TASTING MENU

Barron Point Oyster
Champagne essence, seaweed-watercress salad

Torchon of Foie Gras
Strawberries, balsamic vinegar and crisp prosciutto

Wild Burgundy Escargot
Gruyère gnocchi, fiddlehead fern and bottarga

Red Snapper Steamed with Lemon Verbena
Green tomato chutney and raw tomato vinaigrette

Duck Breast
Pluots, chocolate-peppercorn vinaigrette

Selection of Artisanal Cheeses

Chocolate Tart
Salted caramel, peanut butter and cocoa nib ice cream

DESSERT SIGNATURES

Pumpkin Parfait
Ginger ice cream, maple marshmallow brûlée

Chocolate Tart
Salted caramel, peanut butter and cocoa nib ice cream

Peach Melba
Raspberries and vanilla ice cream

Pineapple Poached in Sauternes
Coconut, cilantro and passion fruit

Selection of Ice Creams and Sorbets

Beat Diabetes approved items in orange.

* See recipe and photo for Halibut Poached in Coconut Milk on pages 256–257.

HALIBUT POACHED IN COCONUT MILK, MUSSELS, CHANTERELLES AND SAFFRON

1 stalk lemongrass, chopped

2 shallots, sliced

2 garlic cloves, crushed

1-inch piece ginger, sliced

2 kaffir lime leaves, chopped

1 tablespoon canola oil

¼ cup white wine

2 14-ounce cans coconut milk

Tiny pinch chile flakes

Salt

½ pint grape or cherry tomatoes

Sugar or a pinch of Splenda

Olive oil

1 pint chanterelle mushrooms, washed

1 garlic clove, crushed

Four 5-6 ounce pieces halibut

1 bunch spinach, leaves picked and washed

Salt

Garlic

BROTH

1. Sauté the lemongrass, shallot, garlic, ginger and lime leaves in the oil until soft.

2. Deglaze with the white wine.

3. Add the coconut milk, chile and salt. Simmer for 30 more minutes.

4. Turn off the flame and allow to infuse for 30 more minutes.

5. Pass through a fine strainer. Season to taste with salt.

VEGETABLES

1. Halve the grape tomatoes and season with a little salt, sugar or Splenda, olive oil and garlic.

2. Spread out on a baking sheet in a single layer.

3. Bake in a preheated 225°F oven for 2 hours.

4. Remove and allow to cool.

5. Heat 4 tablespoons olive oil in a large sauté pan. Add the chanterelle mushrooms and season with salt. Then add a crushed clove of garlic.

6. Continue to cook for 5 minutes. Remove from the pan and allow to drain.

HALIBUT

1. Place the four pieces of halibut in a shallow pan that the fish fit in fairly tightly.

2. Pour the hot coconut broth over the fish and cover the pan.

3. Place in a preheated 350°F oven for 10 minutes, or cook on top of the stove for 10 minutes, but don't allow to boil.

4. Test the fish for doneness with a cake tester or small knife.

5. Heat a sauté pan with 2 tablespoons olive oil, add the chanterelles and cook for 2 minutes. Add the tomatoes and then the spinach. Cook for another 2 minutes, just enough to wilt the spinach.

6. Spoon the mixture into the middle of 4 soup plates.

7. Using a spatula, remove the halibut from the broth and place on top of the vegetables.

8. Spoon a little broth over each piece of fish.

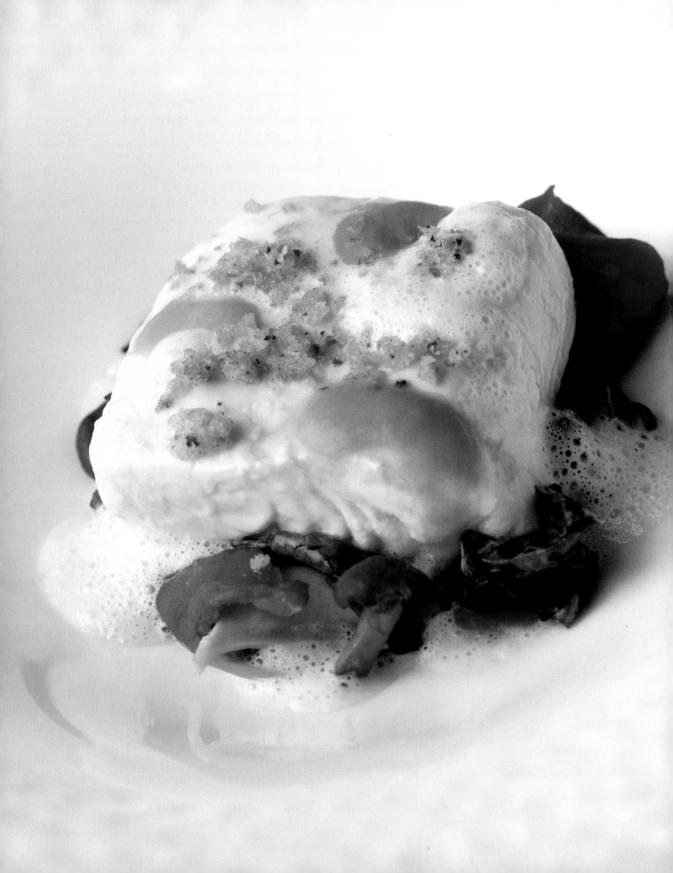

SALAD OF MATSUTAKE MUSHROOMS, PEA GREENS, PINE NUTS AND UBRIACO

4 cups pea shoots

10 matsutake mushrooms (could substitute white mushrooms)

¼ cup pine nuts, toasted

¼ cup picholine (green) olives, cut into quarters

2 tablespoons olive oil

Squeeze of lemon juice

Ubriaco cheese shavings

1. Slice the mushrooms thinly on a mandolin.

2. Combine with the pea shoots, pine nuts and olives in a salad bowl.

3. Toss with the olive oil, lemon juice and a pinch of salt.

4. Arrange on four plates and finish with the Ubriaco cheese on top.

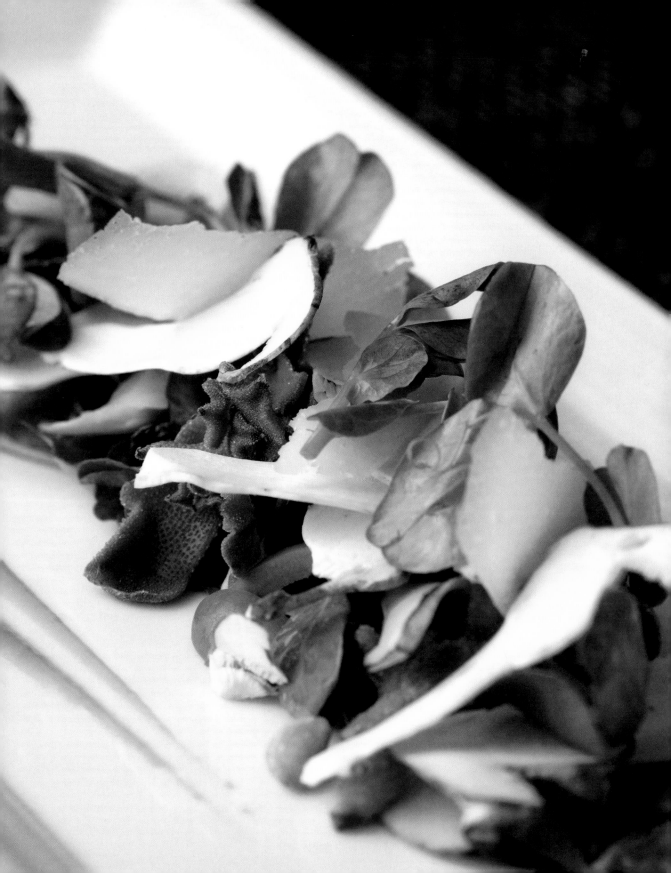

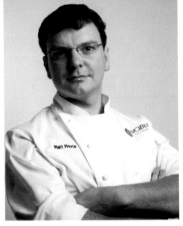

Nobu Chef Matt Hoyle

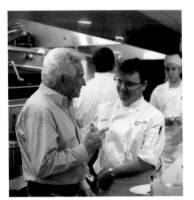

Dr. Shapiro in the kitchen
with Chef Hoyle.

Nobu

Nobu, the world's most recognized Japanese restaurant, known for its innovative new-style Japanese cuisine, started as a business partnership in 1994 between chef Nobu Matsuhisa and his partners actor Robert De Niro, restaurateur Drew Nieporent, producer Meir Teper, and managing partner Richie Notar. With the original restaurant in New York, the Nobu brand is now an empire, with twenty-five restaurants across the globe. Nobu restaurants, all a visual and culinary delight, continue to win unprecedented praise and rave reviews from such publications as the *New York Times,* the *Zagat* surveys, and the *Michelin* guides. The restaurant's perennial popularity and devoted following are a tribute to Nobu putting his own spin on traditional Japanese cooking. For additional information, visit www.noburestaurants.com.

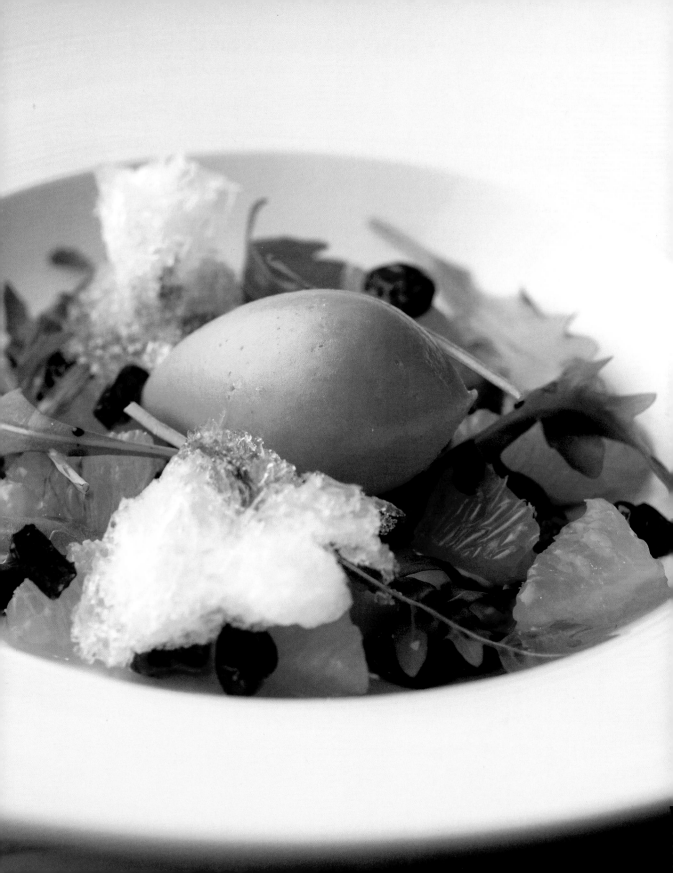

MENU

SPECIAL HOT DISHES

Eggplant with Miso

Sea Urchin Tempura

Rock Shrimp Tempura with Ponzu or Creamy Spicy Sauce

King Crab Tempura with Amazu Ponzu

Mushroom Salad

Squid "Pasta" with Light Garlic Sauce

**Chilean Sea Bass with Black Bean Sauce

Black Cod with Miso

Creamy Spicy Crab

Beef Toban Yaki

COMBINATION LUNCHES

Lobster with Wasabi Pepper Sauce

Scallop or Shrimp with Spicy Garlic Sauce

Arctic Char with Jalapeno Cilantro Sauce

Wild Striped Bass with Shiso Salso

Salmon with Anticucho,
Balsamic Teriyaki or Wasabi Pepper Sauce

Chicken with Anticucho,
Balsamic Teriyaki or Wasabi Pepper Sauce

Ribeye with Anticucho,
Balsamic Teriyaki or Wasabi Pepper Sauce

Tenderloin with Anticucho,
Balsamic Teriyaki or Wasabi Pepper Sauce

DESSERT

*Equilibrium
Fresh oranges, kuromitsu jelly, lemon olive oil, cherry balsamic, cranberries, pecans, fresh arugula with blood orange sorbetto

Tofu "Cheesecake"
Blueberry kanten and frozen champagne mango cream

Mélange
Lychee kanten, raspberry mousse, elderflower snow and peppercorn tuille

Bento Box
Ocumare chocolate fondant cake, sesame crisp with green tea matcha gelato

Alba
Lemon sponge, blood orange ice, black sesame gelato with almond milk soup

Orange-Saffron Cremoso
Pistachio sponge, coconut sorbetto and cardamom tuille

White Peach and Jasmine Soup
Peanut crumble and Nobu beer gelato

Seasonal Fruit Plate

Infused Fruit Nobu Soju
Served chilled

Selection of House-Made Gelati and Sorbetti

Beat Diabetes approved items in orange.

* See photo of Equilibrium on page 261.

** See photo of Chilean Sea Bass with Black Bean Sauce on page 263.

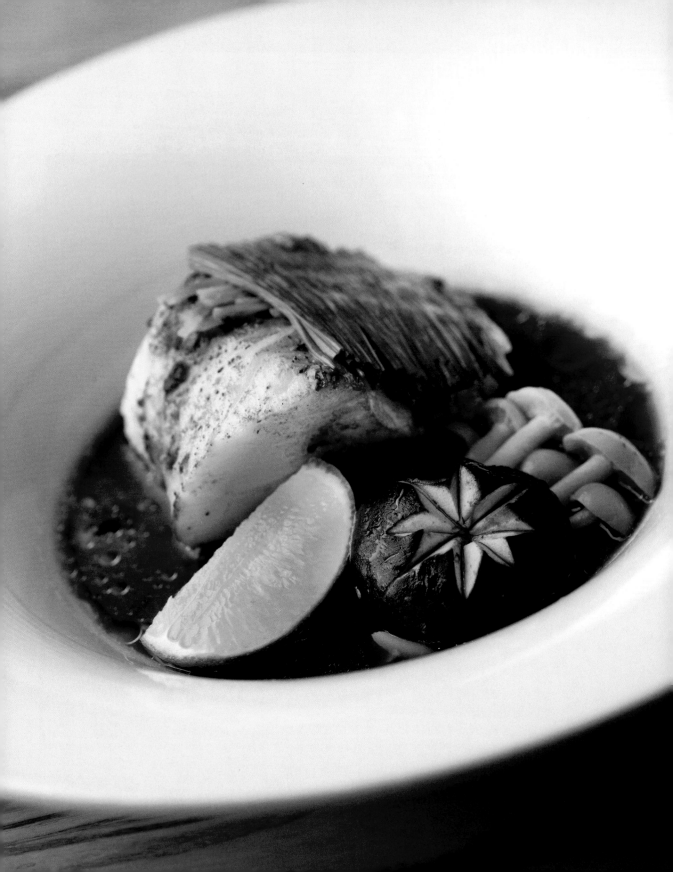

MENU

NOBU SPECIAL COLD DISHES

Bigeye & Bluefin Toro Tartar with Caviar

Salmon or Yellowtail Tartar with Caviar

Sashimi Salad with Matsuhisa Dressing

Lobster Shiitake Salad with Spicy Lemon Dressing

Lobster Inaniwa Pasta Salad

Yellowtail Sashimi with Jalapeño

Fluke Sashimi with Dried Red Miso and Yuzu Sauce

Shiromi Usuzukuri

Tiradito Nobu Style

Salmon Kelp Roll

Bigeye Tuna Tataki with Tosazu

Tomato Ceviche

Ceviche Nobu-Style

NEW-STYLE SASHIMI

Salmon

Kumamoto Oyster

Whitefish

Scallop

SALADS

Edamame

Combination Sunomo

Watercress Rock Shrimp Salad

Field Greens

Oshitashi

Shishito Peppers

*Shiitake Mushroom Salad

Heart of Palm Salad with Jalapeño Dressing

Kelp Salad

Oshinko

SOUPS

Miso

Clam Miso

Akadashi

Mushroom

Clear Soup

Spicy Seafood

Beat Diabetes approved items in orange.

*See photo of Shiitake Mushroom Salad on page 265.

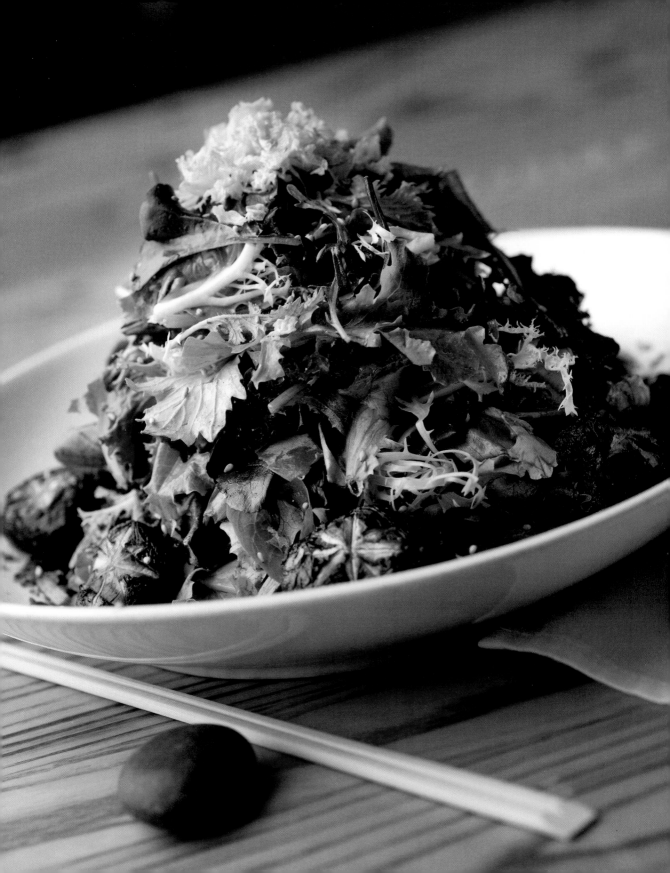

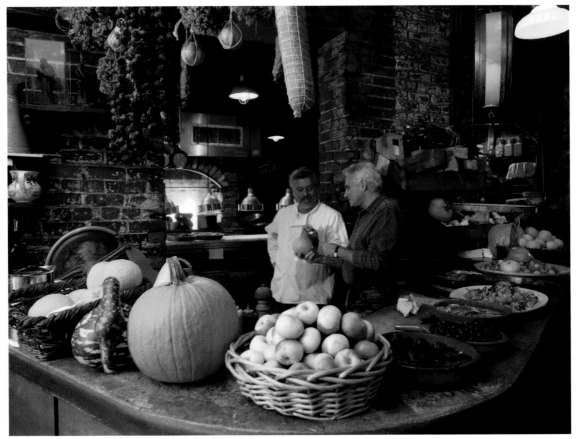

Dr. Shapiro talking to his good friend Frank DeCarlo, chef and owner of Peasant restaurant.

Peasant

Enter one of our favorite restaurants. Peasant's rustic Italian cuisine uses the simplest and freshest ingredients straight from the market. Peasant's philosophy is to go back to the basics, when food was true and beautiful. Grilled whole fish, wood-roasted game, homemade pastas, risotto with the catch of the day and pizzas are all cooked on open fires in an artisanal kitchen, attracting great chefs from all over the world, such as Alain Ducasse, Paul Bocuse and Jean-Louis Palladin as well as New York City's finest, Eric Ripert, Daniel Boulud and Jean-Georges Vongerichten.

Adam Platt from *New York Magazine* writes:

Peasant is exactly right. From its stunningly backlit brick-walled kitchen that features only open-fire cooking to its incredibly appealing pan-Italian menu, chef-owner Frank De Carlo has reason to bust his buttons every night, and you have almost too many reasons to undo a couple of yours. I like the little bowl of sweet ricotta cheese served gratis to the rowdy food scholars in the house, and I'm also partial to the brick-oven-baked rabbit, stewed in cannellini beans with salty strips of pancetta, and the perfectly oval pizza bianca pooled with olive oil.

MENU

SPECIAL HOT DISHES

Zuppa di Ceci
Black chickpea soup

Panzanella
Tuscan bread salad

Acciuga e Radice
Anchovy & radish

Insalata di Tonno
Tuna with white beans

Insalata Stagione
Seasonal vegetable salad

Burrata
Cow's milk cheese with wood-roasted tomatoes

Prosciutto e Frutta
Cured ham & seasonal fruit

Contecchino con Lenticchie
With lentils

Bocconcini
Small balls of mozzarella & speck

Seppie in Terracotta
Cuttlefish, cherry tomatoes and parsley

Sarde al Forno
Sardines, olive oil and bread crumbs

Polpi in Purgatorio
Baby octopus, chile peppers

Trippa alla Fiorentina
Beef tripe

Pizza Margherita D.O.C.
Tomato, basil, mozzarella di bufala

Pizza Peperoncini e Soppressata
Hot chile and dried sausage

Pizza Bianca con Mortadella
Mozzarella, ricotta, parmigiano reggiano and cured pork

Pizza Speck e Rucola
Cured ham & arugula

Spaghetti Vongole
With manila clams & tomatoes

Razza con Capperi
Skate with lemon, white wine and capers

Orata Alla Griglia
Whole grilled sea bass

Beat Diabetes approved items in orange.

SICILIAN TUNA & BEAN SALAD

2 ounces cannellini beans

Salt

1 ounce extra-virgin olive oil

½ lemon, cut into 2 wedges

Small handful of rocket (arugula)

1 ounce red onion, sliced

1 ounce fennel, julienned

1 ounce celery, chopped

3 black gaeta olives

5 ounces of cured tuna in olive oil (preferably from Sicily or Calabria)

Freshly ground pepper

This dish is one of Peasant's specialties.

1. Rinse beans well, place them in a bowl covered with water and soak overnight. Drain beans and place in pot with 1 quart water. Bring to a boil over medium-high heat and then reduce to low. Cover and cook 40 minutes, until tender but not soft. Add salt in last 10 minutes of cooking.

2. Drain beans and transfer to a bowl. Add half the olive oil and a squeeze of lemon wedge. Let cool. Then toss arugula, red onion, fennel, celery and olives with remaining olive oil and a squeeze of lemon. Place on a plate, add beans on top and then place tuna on top of beans. Finish with pepper.

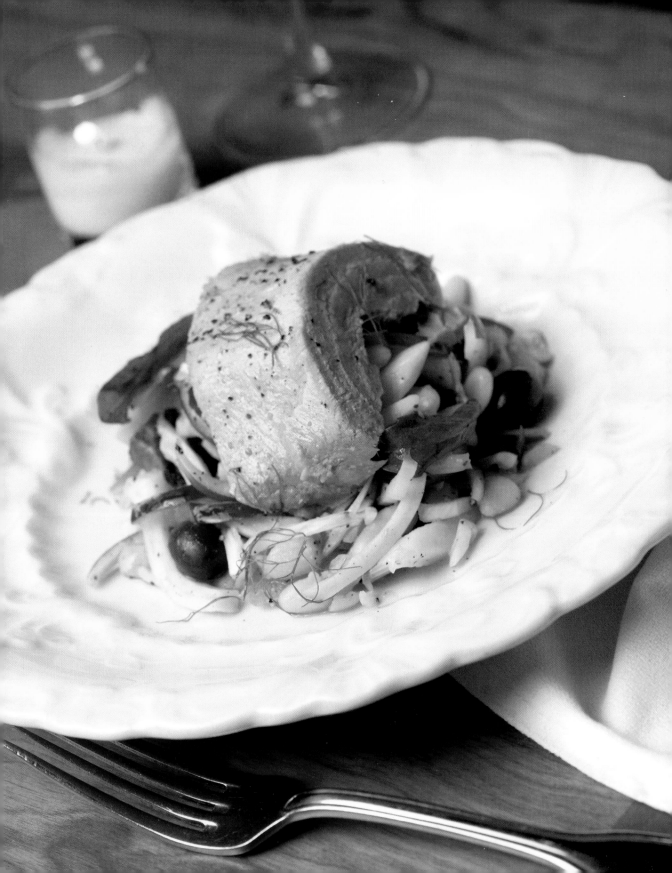

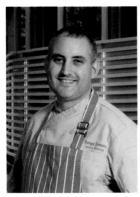

Chef Jeremy Bearman

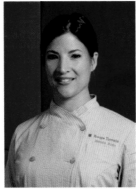

Nutritionist Natalia Rusin

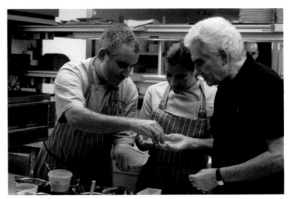

Dr. Shapiro tasting ingredients
in the kitchen at Rouge Tomate.

Rouge Tomate

Located in the heart of midtown Manhattan and recently awarded a Michelin star, Rouge Tomate, designed by award-winning architectural firm Bentel & Bentel, is the ideal destination for after-work cocktails, romantic dinners or a late-night rendezvous. Executive chef Jeremy Bearman, an alumnus of L'Atelier de Joel Robuchon in Las Vegas and New York City's db Bistro Moderne, and culinary nutritionist Natalia Rusin invite you to enjoy their twist on modern American cuisine. A stunning location with rich, natural wood surrounds a seductive bar and lounge, offering the perfect sanctuary from urban chaos. In-house juice bar and specialty cocktails add to this sleek environment. Featuring artwork from Per Fronth, an exposed glass kitchen and cranberry pool, Rouge Tomate offers the best in business, casual and special-event dining.

MENU

APPETIZERS

Freshly Dug Potato and Leek Soup
Farm egg, chive oil and crispy garlic

Market Oysters
Pomegranate mignonette, crispy ginger and cilantro

*Local Fluke Ceviche
Summer melon, avocado, kaffir lime and cilantro

Chickpea Hummus
Sweet peppers, house-cured olives and flatbread crisps

Sauteed Atlantic Calamari
Broccolini, butter beans, brown garlic and smoked paprika

Long Island Duck and Walnut Terrine
Apple-cranberry preserve, pickled celery root, grain mustard and walnut toast

House-Cured Sardines
Heirloom cauliflower, basil pistou, sweet onion and lemon confit

*See recipe and photo for Local Fluke Ceviche on pages 274–275.

MENU

DAILY SPECIAL

Arctic Char "Gravlax"
Apple, daikon radish, celery, ginger oil and trout roe

MARKET SALADS

Brussels Sprout Leaves and Local Pear
Berkshire prosciutto, duchilly hazelnuts, lemon and aged balsamic

Warm Octopus and Summer Bean
Guindilla peppers, arugula, olive and tomato-provençal vinaigrette

Frisée Watercress and Endive Salad
Ewe's milk blue, market grapes, quince paste and walnut vinaigrette

Market Lettuces and Fresh Herbs
Garden sprouts, lemon and extra-virgin olive oil

ENTRÉES

Winter Squash Farrotto
Gala apple, lacinato kale, Parmesan and sage oil

Piedmontese Grass-Fed Flank Steak
Sunburst squash, heirloom eggplant, smoked paprika, cilantro and tomato vinaigrette

Homemade Fettuccine with Wild Mushrooms
Sunchoke, celery root and chervil

Local Shellfish Cioppino
Fennel, fingerling potatoes, saffron and sourdough crostini

Long Island Duck en Sous Vide
Crispy leg, buckwheat crêpe, kohlrabi and huckleberry jus

*Seared Whole Brook Trout with Cauliflower
Heirloom cauliflower, chanterelles, almond and concord grape vinaigrette

Diver Scallops à la Plancha
Goat's milk polenta, brussels sprouts, lobster mushrooms, prosciutto, lemon vinaigrette and mâche

DESSERTS

Concord Grape
Warm praline tart, red & black grapes, concord grape sorbet and hazelnuts

Market Pear
Maple-roasted sweet potato brûlée, cranberry and crystallized ginger

Huckleberry
Warm pistachio crêpes, lemon and house-made ricotta

Medjool Date
Local washed-rind cheese, beldi olives, Asian pear and semolina toast

Banana
Chocolate pudding cake, Earl Grey, feulletine and banana-walnut ice cream

Fall Fruit & Sorbet Plate

Assorted cookie plate

Beat Diabetes approved items in orange.

---

*See recipe and photo for Seared Whole Brook Trout with Cauliflower on pages 272–273.

SEARED WHOLE BROOK TROUT WITH CAULIFLOWER

4 whole brook trout

Sea salt

Cracked pepper

4 ½ teaspoons olive oil

4 cups white cauliflower

2 cups almond milk

7 teaspoons almond oil

4 cups heirloom cauliflower
(1 cup each purple, yellow,
white and romanesco
cauliflower)

4 teaspoons olive oil

¼ cup water

1 cup chanterelle mushrooms

⅓ cup grapes

2 tablespoons almonds

2 teaspoons parsley

1 cup Concord grape juice

1. Remove head and tail of trout if desired. Remove backbone. Season each side with salt and pepper. In a large skillet, heat 2 teaspoons olive oil, and sear each side of fish until cooked through.

2. Put 4 cups white cauliflower and 2 cups almond milk into medium saucepan and cook on medium heat until cauliflower is tender. Remove from heat and puree mixture with 2 teaspoons almond oil. Season to taste with sea salt.

3. Chop heirloom cauliflower into bite-sized florets. Cook each type of cauliflower separately so that colors remain intact. Use ½ teaspoon olive oil in sauté pan with 1 tablespoon water to cook cauliflower until tender.

4. Sauté mushrooms over medium high heat in 2 teaspoons olive oil and season to taste.

5. Slice grapes and almonds and combine with 2 teaspoons almond oil and chopped parsley.

6. Reduce 1 cup of grape juice down to ¼ cup. Whisk in 3 teaspoons almond oil.

7. Just prior to serving, combine heirloom cauliflower and chanterelle mushrooms and distribute evenly over 4 plates. Next place trout over cauliflower and mushrooms. Place cauliflower puree off to side. Top the trout with grape and almond topping. Drizzle Concord grape sauce over plate.

Yield: 4 servings

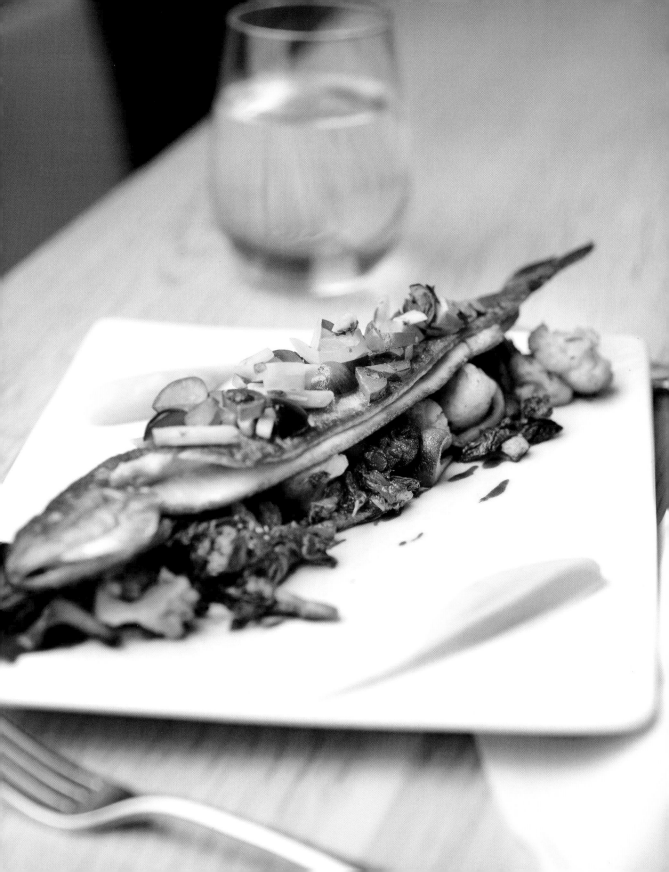

LOCAL FLUKE CEVICHE

12 ounces fluke (sashimi grade), sliced thin

¼ cup thinly sliced red onion

1 jalapeño, julienne

1 tablespoon chopped mint

1 tablespoon chopped cilantro

1 ½ tablespoons fresh lime juice

½ tablespoon extra-virgin olive oil

¼–½ teaspoon sea salt

3 tablespoons each of several varieties of melon (watermelon, cantaloupe, honeydew), small cubes

20 pieces air-popped popcorn

1. **Slice fluke and mix with onion, jalapeño, herbs, lime juice, olive oil and salt. Divide mixture into 4 equal parts and place fluke on 4 plates. Garnish each plate with melon and popcorn. Serve immediately.**

Yield: 4 servings

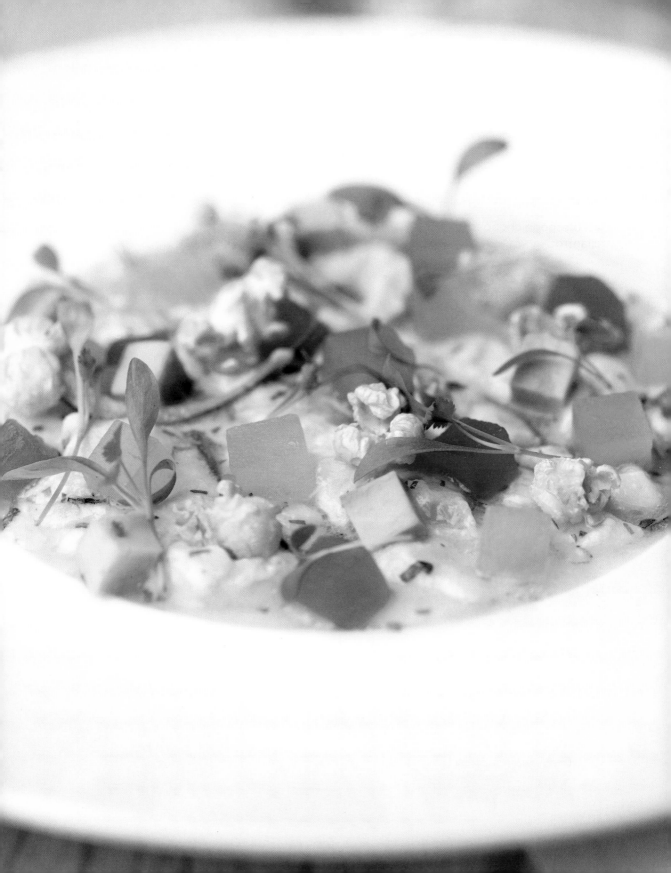

Here are some more menus from a few of our other favorite places to eat in New York.

Dawat Haute Cuisine of India

MENU

STARTERS

Baghari Jhinga
Succulent shrimp, flavored with garlic, mustard seeds and curry leaves

SOUPS & SALAD

Ginger Cauliflower Soup
A silken pureed spicy ginger-flavored soup

Mulligatawny Soup
A spicy favorite of Anglo-India, made with split peas, vegetables and chicken

Healthy Sprouted Bean Salad
Bean sprouts, cucumber, carrot and sweet pepper salad

Dawat Kachumber Salad
Mixed greens, cucumber, tomato salad topped with sliced almonds and raisins along with chef's special dressing

KEBABS

Vegetable "Seekh" Kebab
Delicately spiced skewered vegetable rolls

TANDOOR (CLAY OVEN) FAVORITES

Tandoori Shrimp
King-size shrimp marinated in mild spices

Chilean Sea Bass Tikka
Chunk of Chilean sea bass, marinated in an aromatic herb mixture

Tandoori Chicken
Chicken marinated in yogurt and mild spices

Chicken Tikka
Boneless chunks of chicken, marinated in yogurt and mild spices

Murgh Jehangiri
Chicken pieces marinated in yogurt with lavish bastings of chili and coriander

Raan
A whole, small tender leg of lamb braised with ginger and whole spices, then roasted in the tandoor oven until it is crisp outside and meltingly tender inside

Whole Tandoori Fish
Whole seasonal fish marinated in yogurt and flavored with dill-like carom seeds before it is roasted

SEAFOOD

Scallops Caldin
Crusty scallops with a green coriander chili sauce—a Goan specialty

Fish in a Mustard Sauce
Chunks of fish in a spicy sauce of crushed mustard seeds and mustard oil

Kerala-Style Konju Pappaas
Shrimp in a coconut sauce, flavored with aromatic curry leaves and smoked tamarind

Parsi-Style Patra-ni-Machhi
Salmon smothered in a fresh coriander chutney, wrapped in a banana leaf and steamed, served with basmati rice

Shrimp Bhuna
Shrimp cooked in specially prepared herbs and spices with a touch of garlic and ginger

MENU

POPULAR CURRIES

Shrimp Curry with Roasted Spices
A delicious shrimp curry, which is both rich and aromatic

Goan Fish Curry
A traditional fish curry from Goa, red hot and delicious

Lamb Curry
A classic dish from northern India

Mughlai Chicken Curry
Chicken cooked with lots of Indian spices and condiments in a rich gravy

Home-Style Chicken Curry
All-time favorite—chicken, fresh ginger, onion and tomato gravy

Vegetable Curry
Mixed vegetables mildly spiced

VEGETARIAN SPECIALTIES

Paneer Makhani
Fresh homemade cheese, folded into creamy tomato sauce

Sauteed Shiitake Mushrooms
Flavored with fresh curry leaves and green coriander

Smoked Eggplant Bharta
Roasted pureed eggplant, ginger, onions, tomatoes and fresh coriander

Mattar Paneer
Fresh homemade cheese cubes cooked with green peas

Saag Paneer
Fresh homemade cheese cubes in a spicy spinach sauce

Baked Eggplant
Thin slices of eggplant coated with a mild sweet-and-sour tamarind sauce and baked

Maharashtrian-Style Farasvi Bhaji
Green beans cooked with freshly grated coconut

Labdharay Aloo
Potatoes with ginger and tomatoes in a thick sauce

Malai Kofta
Mixed vegetable croquette in a savory, spicy sauce

Tadka Dal
Slow-simmered matpe beans and red kidney beans, sautéed with tomatoes, ginger, cumin and onion

Yellow Dal
Mildly flavored yellow split lentils sautéed with onions, ginger and spices

Vegetable Jal Frazie
Mixed vegetables with cottage cheese, mildly spiced

Zeera Aloo
Spicy potatoes flavored with whole and ground cumin seeds

Sindhi Karhi
A specialty of the community of western India, vegetarian stew made with chickpea flour and vegetables and seasoned with tamarind and fenugreek seeds

Sarson Ka Saag
Fresh mustard greens and spinach cooked in a Punjabi village style

VEGAN

Bhindi Masala
Okra blended with browned onions and dried mango

Bhuni Gobhi
Cauliflower stir-fried with ginger and cumin seeds

Channa Masala
A spicy chickpea preparation

Beat Diabetes **approved items in orange.**

Marea

MENU

E PER COMINCIARE (ITEMS TO BE SHARED BY THE TABLE)

Ricci
Sea urchin, lardo and sea salt

Sardine
House-marinated sardines, arugula

Melanzane
Eggplant and sepia arancini

Zeppole
Seaweed, shrimp and chickpea fritters

CRUDO AL TAGLIO (SLICED RAW FISH AND SHELLFISH)

Passera
Long Island fluke, lemon thyme and Ligurian olive oil

Tonno
Bigeye tuna, oyster crema and crispy artichokes

Seppia
Cuttlefish tagliatelle, soffrito crudo and bottarga di muggine

Pesce Volante
Flying fish, sea beans and citrus oil

Astice
Nova Scotia lobster, sun-dried tomatoes, olives and plum

Sparnocchi
Alaksan spot prawns and lava salt

Dentice
Pacific snapper, whole-wheat panzanella

Pesce Sventola
North Carolina blowfish, Pugliese oil

Vongole
Geoduck clam, fresh chiles and lemon

Cannolicchi
Marinated razor clams, fennel and peperoncino

Capesante
Scallop, orange, wild fennel and arugula

Lancia
Blue marlin, sturgeon caviar and mussels vinaigrette

Polipo
Octopus, chili oil, lemon and parsley

Sgombro
Pacific jack mackerel, duck prosciutto and pomegranate

Scampi
Pacific langoustines and Murray River pink salt

Ventresca
Bigeye toro tartare, Ligurian olivada, fried capers

ASSAGGIO DI TRE — TASTING OF THREE CRUDO

Ostriche East and West Coast oysters with morellino mignonette and cucumber-lemon vinegar	Pemaquid	Hog Island	Dennis
	Maine	California	Massachusetts
	Beausoleil	Wellfleet	Tomahawk
	New Brunswick	Massachusetts	New York

Beat Diabetes **approved items in orange.**

MENU

ANTIPASTI (SEASONAL APPETIZERS)

Granchio
Blue crab, grilled watermelon, castelvetrano olives and mint

Tartare
Hawaiian blue prawns, chanterelles and marcona almonds

Astice
Nova Scotia lobster, burrata, eggplant al funghetto and basil

Polipo
Grilled octopus, Sicilian couscous, pine nuts and apricot mostarda

Zuppa
Lobster and butternut squash soup, porcini mushrooms and lobster butter

Ricciola
Lightly cooked yellowtail, tendon coppa, pine mushroom and radicchio

Calamari
Shrimp ripieno, controne beans, cavolo nero and squid ink

Baccala
Housemade salt cod, heirloom tomatoes and watercress

Uovo
Slow-poached egg, monkfish cheeks, wild mushrooms and garlic chips

SECONDI DI PESCE (SEASONAL FISH DISHES)

San Pietro
Sautéed John Dory, marinated salsify, roasted Brussels sprouts, fresh pancetta and saba

Spada
Grilled Hawaiian swordfish, delicate squash, dandelion greens, cara cara oranges and pistachios

Ippoglosso
Seared Alaskan halibut, beluga lentils, cipollini agrodolce and broccoli rabe

Capesante
Porcini dusted sea scallops, braised leeks, celery root, soppressata and crustacean sugetto

Brodetto di Pesce
Adriatic seafood soup, clams, langoustine, scallop, spot prawns and bass

Seppia
Grilled Mediterranean cuttlefish, braised escarole, taggia olives, Livornese sauce and wild oregano

INTERI WHOLE FISH AND SHELLFISH

Rombo
Turbot, roasted

Sogliola
Dover sole, sautéed

Branzino
Wild bass, salt baked

Scampi
Langoustines, seared

CONDIMENTI (SAUCES)

Salmoriglio
Sicilian caper, wild oregano

Livornese
Tomato, olive and caper

Limone
Citrus lemon

Salsa Verde
Parsley, basil

CONTORNI (SIDE DISHES)

Braised Escarole, Anchovy

Fingerling Potatoes, Rosemary

Eggplant Agrodolce

Roasted Brussels Sprouts, Pancetta

Wild Arugula and Lemon

Roasted Beets, Ricotta Salata

Rosa Mexicano

MENU

DINNER ENTRADAS

Guacamole en Molcajete
Freshly made guacamole with avocado, jalapeño, tomato, onion and cilantro, served with warm corn tortillas, tortilla chips, salsa pasilla de Oaxaca and salsa de tomatillo y habanero

Ensalada de la Casa/Field Greens Salad
Mixed field greens, shredded jicama, carrots and cherry tomatoes dressed in a pomegranate vinaigrette

Ceviche de Atun y Camarones/Marinated Seafood
Chilled citrus-marinated tuna and shrimp

Ensalada de Vegetales à la Parilla/Grilled Vegetable Salad
Zucchini, hearts of palm, artichokes, corn and chile-rubbed red bliss potatoes tossed in a roasted tomato-oregano vinaigrette

ENCHILADAS

Mole de Xico/Beef
Two soft corn tortillas filled with shredded chipotle beef, topped with Veracruz mole made with raisins, plantains, hazelnuts, pine nuts and mulato, ancho and pasila chiles, garnished with crema and queso fresco

Suizas/Chicken
Two soft corn tortillas filled with pulled roasted chicken, topped with a creamy tomatillo sauce and melted Chihuahua cheese

Rancheras/Vegetable
Two soft corn tortillas filled with wild mushrooms and spinach topped with a mild Mexican tomato sauce, garnished with crema and queso fresco

Jaiba/Jumbo Lump Crab
Two soft corn tortillas filled with jumbo lump crabmeat, topped with a creamy tomatillo sauce, melted Chihuahua cheese and pumpkin seeds

PLATILLOS PRINCIPALES

All entrees are served with family-style rice, refried black beans and two condiment salsas: Pasillo de Oaxaca and Salsa de Tomatillo y Habanero

Ensalada con Atun/Tuna Salad
Avocado leaf-crusted seared rare tuna, served on a crispy black bean tostada over jicama, mango, cabbage slaw with mixed field greens and tropical fruit salsa

Alambre de Camarones/Shrimp Brochette
Grilled shrimp marinated in a garlic vinaigrette over house rice with onions, tomatoes, serrano peppers and roasted tomato-jalapeño-caper sauce

Mariposa de Huachinango/Red Snapper
Pan-roasted whole buttterflied red snapper, brushed with guajillo chile and served with roasted tomatillo and garlic molcajete salsa

Salmon e Manchamenteles/Salmon Filet with Tropical Fruit Mole
Grilled organic salmon over black beans with zucchini and roasted corn, served over a mole of ancho chiles and tropical fruits

Beat Diabetes approved items in orange.

You can find delicious, healthful meals to help beat diabetes in restaurants outside of New York, too. Just take a look at what to order off these partial menus at some of our other favorite establishments across the country.

California Pizza Kitchen

MENU

APPETIZERS

Cabo Crab Cakes
Pan-sautéed blue crab cakes served with roasted corn and black bean salsa and a roasted red pepper aioli

Tuscan Hummus
Tuscan white beans puréed with sesame, garlic, lemon and spices, garnished with Italian parsley, fresh Roma tomatoes, basil and garlic, served with warm pizza-pita bread

Lettuce Wraps
Minced chicken and/or shrimp, wok-seared with shiitake mushrooms, water chestnuts and green onions in a soy-ginger sauce, served on a bed of crispy rice noodles with a side of spicy chili-ginger sauce

SOUPS

Asparagus Soup
A creamless vegetarian soup garnished with garlic-herb croutons

Adobe Chicken Chowder
A creamy rich chowder with chicken, Wehani rice, sweet roasted corn, green chilies, mild onions, bell peppers and cilantro, topped with crispy corn tortilla strips

Dakota Smashed Pea and Barley Soup
Hearty, vegetarian split pea with barley, carrots, onions and savory herbs, garnished with chopped green onions

Sedona Tortilla Soup
Vine-ripened tomatoes, tomatillos and corn with mild green chilies and Southwestern spices, garnished with crispy corn tortilla strips

SALADS

Grilled Vegetable Salad
Grilled asparagus, Japanese eggplant, zucchini, green onions and roasted corn served warm over a bed of chilled Romaine lettuce, fresh avocado and sun-dried tomatoes in a Dijon balsamic vinaigrette

Miso Salad
Shredded Napa cabbage with fresh avocado, julienne cucumbers, daikon, edamame, carrots, red cabbage, green onions, cilantro, crispy rice noodles and crispy wontons tossed in a miso dressing and topped with blue crab and shrimp

SPECIALTIES

Ginger Salmon
Pan-sautéed Atlantic salmon topped with chopped cilantro, green onions and a sweet ginger sauce, **served with wok-stirred Mandarin noodles,** snow peas and sesame seeds and wok-stirred mixed vegetables

Pan-Sautéed Salmon
Lightly seasoned Atlantic salmon, served with fresh grilled asparagus and spaghettini in a creamy lemon-caper sauce or wok-stirred mixed vegetables (served blackened upon request)

Chili's

MENU

GUILTLESS GRILL

Guiltless Cedar Plank Tilapia
Seasoned tilapia fillet topped with house-made pico de gallo and a lime wedge, cooked and served on a cedar plank

Guiltless Black Bean Burger
Meatless black bean patty topped with low-fat ranch on a wheat bun, served with lettuce, tomato, onion and pickle

Grilled Shrimp Alfredo
Spicy garlic-and-lime-grilled shrimp over penne pasta tossed in creamy Alfredo sauce, topped with diced tomatoes, green onions and Parmesan cheese and served with garlic toast

Grilled Salmon with Garlic and Herbs
Salmon fillet seasoned with garlic and herbs, served with rice and seasonal veggies

NOT JUST SIDES

Loaded Mashed Potatoes

Homestyle Fries

Mashed Potatoes with Black Pepper Gravy

Black Beans

Rice

Sweet Corn on the Cob

Seasonal Veggies

Cinnamon Apples

BOWL FULL OF FLAVOR

Chili or Soup and Side Salad
A delicious bowl of chili or soup with a Caesar or house side salad

Soups of the Day

SALADS

Spicy Garlic-and-Lime-Grilled Shrimp Salad
Spicy garlic-and-lime-grilled shrimp, mixed cheese, corn relish, house-made pico de gallo and crispy tortilla strips, topped with cilantro, served with fire-roasted tomato vinaigrette

Beat Diabetes approved items in orange.

Denny's

MENU

BREAKFAST

Veggie-Cheese Omelette
Three-egg omelette with green peppers, onions and mushrooms folded in with diced tomatoes and shredded Cheddar cheese (order with egg whites and no cheese)

Hearty Wheat Pancakes
Three hearty wheat pancakes (order with sugar-free syrup)

Bacon Strips (Four)

Turkey Bacon Strips (Four)

Sausage Links (Four)

Chicken Sausage Patties (Two)

Grilled Honey Ham Slice

Egg Whites

Hash Browns

Cheddar Cheese Hash Browns

Everything Hash Browns

Buttermilk Pancakes

Hearty Wheat Pancakes

Toast

Pancake Puppies

Bagel and Cream Cheese

Biscuit

English Muffin

Grits

Oatmeal

Granola

Seasonal Fruit

DINNER – Includes choice of a bowl of soup or a garden salad

Grilled Shrimp Skewer
One skewer of succulent shrimp grilled and placed over savory vegetable rice pilaf, served with choice of one side and dinner bread

Homestyle Meatloaf
One slice of classic meatloaf, grilled and covered in brown gravy, served with choice of two sides and dinner bread

Grilled Chicken
Delicious, seasoned grilled chicken breast, served with choice of two sides and dinner bread

Senior Country-Fried Steak

BURGERS

Boca Burger
A meatless combination of soy, spices and cheese, served with lettuce, tomato, pickles and red onions

SOUPS

Bowl of Soup
Soups are kettle-cooked to be rich and hearty

AMERICAN DINNER CLASSICS

Lemon-Pepper Grilled Tilapia
A seasoned whitefish filet grilled and topped with a tangy lemon-pepper butter sauce (sauce on side), served on a bed of savory vegetable rice pilaf with choice of two sides and dinner bread

Tilapia Ranchero
A seasoned whitefish filet grilled and topped with freshly made pico de gallo and diced avocado, served with a side of creamy ranchero mashed potatoes and dinner bread

DINNER SIDE CHOICES

Coleslaw	Fiesta Corn	Mashed Potatoes	Smoked Cheddar Mashed Potatoes
Corn	French Fries	Onion Rings	
Country-Fried Potatoes	Green Beans	Ranchero Mashed Potatoes	Tomato Slices
Dippable Veggies	Hash Browns		Vegetable Rice Pilaf

Olive Garden

MENU

ANTIPASTI (APPETIZERS)

Mussels di Napoli
Mussels in the shell, simmered with wine, garlic butter and onions

Sicilian Scampi
Large shrimp sautéed in extra-virgin olive oil with white wine, garlic and lemon

ZUPPE E INSALATE (SOUPS AND SALADS)

Minestrone
Fresh vegetables, beans and pasta in a light tomato broth

Garden-Fresh Salad
Famous house salad, tossed with signature Italian dressing

PESCE (FISH AND SEAFOOD)

Shrimp Primavera
Shrimp, bell peppers, onions and mushrooms in a bold arrabbiata sauce over penne

Herb-Grilled Salmon
Salmon filet brushed with Italian herbs and extra-virgin olive oil, served with seasoned broccoli

Grilled Shrimp Caprese
Grilled marinated shrimp served over angel hair pasta with melted mozzarella, fresh basil and tomatoes in a garlic-butter sauce

Seafood Alfredo
Sautéed shrimp and scallops tossed with creamy fettuccine Alfredo

Parmesan Crusted Tilapia
Oven-baked delicate whitefish crusted with Parmesan cheese, served with Italian vegetables over angel hair tossed in a light garlic-butter sauce

Shrimp and Asparagus Risotto
Large sautéed shrimp served over creamy Parmesan risotto with asparagus

Seafood Portofino
Mussels, scallops, shrimp and mushrooms with linguine in a garlic-butter wine sauce

POLLO E PESCE (CHICKEN AND SEAFOOD)

Venetian Apricot Chicken
Grilled chicken breast in an apricot citrus sauce, served with broccoli, asparagus and diced tomatoes

Shrimp Primavera
Shrimp, bell peppers, onions and mushrooms in a bold arrabbiata sauce over penne

Beat Diabetes **approved items in orange.**

Outback Steakhouse

MENU

APPETIZERS

Seared Ahi Tuna

SALADS

Dressings—Tangy Tomato Dressing (fat-free), Vinegar

Fresh Lemon or Olive Oil and Red Wine Vinegar

House Salad (order without croutons)

Caesar Salad (order without croutons)

Queensland Salad (order without croutons)

Entrée Caesar Salad (order without croutons)

ADD-ONS AND SIDES

Fresh Steamed French Green Beans

Fresh Seasonal Veggies

Jacket Potato

Sweet Potato

ENTRÉES

Shrimp and Veggie Griller
(order without butter or glaze during preparation)

Salmon
(order prepared without butter or seasoning; with fresh seasonal veggies without butter)

STRAIGHT FROM THE SEA

Atlantic Salmon

Lobster Tail

Ruby Tuesday

MENU

APPETIZERS

Jumbo Lump Crab Cake
Almost all crab and nearly no cake, made from fresh, premium jumbo lump crab meat and seared to a golden brown

PREMIUM SEAFOOD

Herb Crusted Tilapia
Tender, mild tilapia crusted with panko garlic bread crumbs **topped with lemon-butter sauce,** with fresh steamed broccoli and brown-rice pilaf

Chesapeake Catch
Spicy, broiled tilapia crowned with a jumbo lump crab cake **and topped with Parmesan cream sauce,** with fresh steamed broccoli and brown-rice pilaf

New Orleans Seafood
Spicy, broiled tilapia topped with sautéed shrimp **and rich Parmesan cream sauce,** served with fresh steamed broccoli and brown-rice pilaf

Parmesan Shrimp Pasta
Tender, spicy shrimp are seasoned and sautéed, then served over pasta in Parmesan cream sauce and accented with diced tomatoes

Asian Glazed Salmon
Grilled Atlantic salmon glazed with a peanut-barbecue sauce to give it a sweet and spicy kick, served with fresh steamed broccoli and brown-rice pilaf

HANDCRAFTED BURGERS

Veggie Burger
Blended with six all-natural garden veggies, long-grain rice and black beans, **topped with Swiss cheese**

Jumbo Lump Crab Burger
Fresh, tender, premium crab cakes, seared to a golden brown, accented with sweet and spicy chili sauce

Blackened Fish
A flaky, tender tilapia fillet, seasoned with Creole spices and broiled, finished with a sweet and spicy chili sauce

SIGNATURE SIDES

Sautéed Baby Portobello Mushrooms	Fresh Steamed Broccoli	Creamy Mashed Cauliflower	Brown-Rice Pilaf
Premium Baby Green Beans	Baked Potato	**White Cheddar Mashed Potatoes**	**Loaded Baked Potato**

Beat Diabetes approved items in orange.

THE SKINNY ON SUPPLEMENTS

Did you know that an estimated 80 percent of Americans use dietary supplements? We do so because we think the supplements will keep us healthy, prevent disease, treat or heal or cure a condition or sickness we have or all of the above.

Supplements embrace a range of possible substances and can include plant extracts, enzymes, vitamins, minerals, fatty acids and more. They are regulated under the Dietary Supplement Health and Education Act of 1994 (DSHEA), but they are generally not subjected to the same rigorous testing as prescription drugs, and neither their safety nor their efficacy need to be established. In other words, let the buyer beware: there is simply no guarantee that the supplement you're using works or that it won't cause some side effect that might itself be harmful.

That is why for anyone and everyone—but especially for diabetics—it is essential that you **always consult your health care provider before taking any supplement.**

Still, many diabetics use supplements to lower their blood sugar or to reduce the risk or the severity of complications from the disease. The use of supplements is widespread and varied, so for purposes of talking about them, we're going to set an agenda of five categories:

- Six popular supplements
- Chromium picolinate, which is controversial
- Vitamins and minerals
- Phytosterols and phytostanols
- Green tea capsules

The following six popular supplements have been particularly sought after by diabetics, and although all have shown some benefits in terms of blood sugar regulation, the testing for specific safety and efficacy concerns has thus far been inadequate. Some have tested safe and free of side effects, some not. Some have been proven effective, some not. So while we can't say all are unsafe or none are effective, we recommend none of them for diabetics. The six are:

- Aloe
- Bitter melon
- Fenugreek
- Ginseng
- Gymnema
- Nopal

Chromium supplementation in the form of chromium picolinate is widely used by diabetics—and widely recommended for them. Chromium is classed as an ultra-trace mineral, which means that it is found in the body in very small amounts—typically measured in micrograms—yet it performs a couple of essential roles in metabolism. Where diabetics in particular are concerned, chromium does seem to enhance insulin action and may thereby help regulate glucose and triglyceride metabolism in type 2 diabetes. Also on the plus side is the fact that chromium deficiency results in insulin resistance and can cause certain lipid abnormalities; these can all be reversed with the use of chromium supplements.

In fact, several studies have shown that using from 100 to 500 mcg of chromium twice a day improved diabetes control, and many experts recommend at least 200 mcg per day for optimal blood sugar regulation.

But some of these studies have been questioned on the grounds that the test subjects may have been chromium deficient to begin with. A number of the studies, in fact, were done in China, where there is believed to be a higher incidence of chromium deficiency than elsewhere, particularly Western countries. And in yet another recent study, a program of chromium supplementation over the course of twelve weeks showed no effect at all on glucose concentration, glucose-regulating hormones or any other measure of glucose metabolism. No wonder the American Diabetes Association, for one, declares that evidence demonstrating the benefit of chromium supplementation is "inconclusive."

Bottom line on chromium? If your body is deficient in this substance to begin with, your diabetes control may well improve with supplements. How do you know whether or not you're deficient? It's hard to establish. And since the amount of chromium present in food varies widely, the best course of action may be to give chromium supplements a try—after checking with your doctor, of course. We recommend a trial dose of 200 mcg per day for one month; if there is no improvement in your blood sugar control, discontinue the supplement. Excess chromium supplementation can lead to toxicity, which in turn may cause skin lesions, gastric ulcers and even liver and kidney impairment. Interestingly, there are no reports of chromium toxicity from food—only from supplements.

Where vitamins and minerals are concerned, we do recommend a basic one-a-day multi-vitamin and mineral supplement. There are two reasons for this recommendation. First, even though eating the Pyramid way is healthy in every respect and provides an ample supply of nutrients, a little added insurance—an extra margin of safety—can't hurt, especially on those days when we may perhaps forget our daily portion of leafy greens!

Second, vitamins B_6 and B_{12} along with folic acid may reduce the levels of a substance in the blood called homocystine, which is associated with cardiovascular disease. Since cardiovascular risk is of particular concern among diabetics, making sure you get those nutrients is important, and about the easiest way to be sure is to take a multivitamin, which invariably contains the recommended daily amount of all three: B_6, B_{12} and folic acid.

Plant sterols and plant stanols—phytosterols and phytostanols—are useful if your total or LDL cholesterol is high. In fact, if that is the case, we recommend them. These substances are extracted from plants—often from soybeans or pine trees—and they work by inhibiting the absorption of cholesterol. They come in tablets or capsules and are available in health stores and pharmacies. We recommend 2 to 3 grams of phytosterols and/or phytostanols a day. You'll find them easy to tolerate, and they can lower your cholesterol by anywhere from 9 percent to 20 percent. (Note: Cholesterol-lowering agents—whether by prescription or over-the-counter—are not recommended during pregnancy.)

Green tea is described as having thermogenic and fat-oxidizing properties—fancy words for burning fat to the tune of 90 calories a day. Do the math: that translates to nearly 10 pounds a year. Green tea has also been found to reduce fasting plasma glucose significantly in type 2 diabetics. And it can reduce the risk of developing coronary heart disease. How? It helps lower both total and LDL cholesterol, and it protects HDL cholesterol against oxidation. In other words, green tea can help prevent type 2 diabetes by decreasing body fat, can help control diabetes by lowering blood sugar and can decrease the risk and severity of diabetes' main complication, coronary heart disease. And if that's not enough, green tea also lowers the risk of many cancers.

Convinced? Take about 400 mg of green tea two to three times a day—or as your doctor recommends.

Our final recommendation is a weight-loss formula developed by Dr. Shapiro called Slenda Rx. This supplement is widely available, and we recommend that it be taken with a full glass of water an hour before each meal. It is composed of four ingredients: glucomannan, green tea, caffeine and hoodia.

1. **Glucomannan.** A 2005 study at the Rush University in Chicago suggests that this soluble fiber (derived from the Asian konjac plant) helps promote feelings of fullness. In fact, the study showed that patients who took glucomannan before each meal lost an average of 5.5 pounds over eight weeks—without any additional dietary changes
2. **Green tea.** Green tea has been proven study after study, to help you burn fat through its thermogenic and fat-oxidizing properties.
3. **Caffeine.** Caffeine also helps suppress your appetite, and acts in conjunction with green tea to provide thermogenesis.

4. **Hoodia.** This ancient, rare botanical has been used for centuries by the San Bushmen of Kalahari Desert. The Bushmen, who live off the land, cut off part of the hoodia stem and eat it to ward off hunger and thirst during nomadic hunting trips. Scientific studies have noted what the Bushmen know—research has isolated several compounds in South African hoodia that help suppress appetite.

SOME OF OUR FAVORITE TOOLS TO BEAT DIABETES

Here are some of our favorite products, used liberally in the demonstrations and recipes throughout this book. Find them at your local supermarket, fine foods market or health food store.

BREADS AND CEREALS	
Arnold—Light 100% Whole Wheat Bread	Tumaro's—Low in Carbs Gourmet Tortillas
Damascus Bakeries—Flax Roll-ups	Kellogg's—All-Bran Extra Fiber
Weight Watchers—English muffins, pita and sliced breads	General Mills—Fiber One
La Tortilla Factory—Low-Carb Tortillas	McCann's—Steel Cut Oats

SOY VEGGIE PRODUCTS	
Marukome—Japan's largest producer of miso	Tofurkey—Beer Brats, kielbasa and Italian sausage
Morningstar Farms—breakfast sausage patties and Meal Starters Recipe Crumbles	Synergia—Bleu cheese and tomato-garlic feta
Yves—meatless Canadian bacon and veggie pepperoni slices	Galaxy Nutritional Foods—American- and cheddar-flavor soy slices
Lightlife—turkey and bologna-style veggie slices	Whole Foods Soy Protein Powder

FROZEN TREATS	
Tofutti—Chocolate Fudge Treats	The Enlightened Gourmet—Absolutely Free Double Chocolate Fudge Swirl
Unilever—Fudgsicles (no sugar added)	Edy's—Fruit Bars (no sugar added)

THE OTHER ESSENTIAL HEALTH CHOICE: EXERCISE

It isn't just poor choices in eating that are responsible for the surge of type 2 diabetes in the United States. Equally defining is the sedentary lifestyle—the sheer inactivity—of far too many Americans. The National Health Interview Survey tells us that fewer than a third of all adults in the United States spend the recommended thirty minutes a day in physical activity, while nearly 40 percent of us aren't active at all.

For diabetics trying to manage their disease, exercise isn't just a recommendation; it's a necessity. *It helps both control the disease and reduce the risk of complications—or the severity of complications if and when they do occur. For those in a prediabetic state, exercise can help delay the onset of the disease or prevent it altogether.*

If you're trying to manage your type 2 diabetes now, here are just some of the benefits regular exercise can bring to you:

- An improved lipid profile—decreased LDL cholesterol and possibly increased HDL cholesterol
- Decreased blood clot formation
- Improved insulin sensitivity
- Decreased body fat—especially intra-abdominal fat
- An improved mental outlook

No wonder the *American Diabetes Association recommends that all people with diabetes get a minimum of 150 minutes of moderate-intensity aerobic exercise weekly.* What is moderate-intensity aerobic exercise? It's exercise where you're working a little—enough to get your heart going. Walking at a brisk pace, cycling on mostly level terrain, raking leaves, shoveling snow: all of these qualify as moderate-intensity aerobic exercise. And here's the real bonus: this kind of aerobic exercise, done regularly, can actually decrease insulin requirements by as much as 100 percent for type 2 diabetics!

But the aerobics are not enough. Type 2 diabetics also need to perform some resistance training three times a week, unless other health conditions or complications make such exercise unadvisable. You don't need to buy fancy weights or barbells, although these work well. All sorts of weight-bearing exercise work—including house cleaning, carrying groceries, dancing and even gardening. The idea is to work against gravity.

Combine the aerobic and the resistance exercises into one workout, polish it off with some stretching and you will help not just your diabetes but your heart and your overall health as well. Of course, always check with your doctor about the type, frequency and intensity of exercise you're doing. Find out also whether you need to monitor your glucose before and after exercise, and whether or how to coordinate exercise with food intake and medications. Your doctor will be glad to help with your exercise regimen. He or she knows that *by undertaking a regular program of exercise and changing their eating habits, three-fourths of today's diabetic patients could safely stop using medications.* Indeed, they'd be better off for it.

LAST WORD

We started this book by offering some pretty scary statistics about diabetes. It almost made it sound as if we were all caught up in a race to stay one step ahead of this killer disease.

It's true. We are in a race. What we've provided you here are the tools you need to win that race. Think of the information we've provided as your racing equipment—the swiftest gear, the fastest shoes. Think of the Beat Diabetes Pyramid as the course of training that will ensure you get to the finish line way ahead of the disease that's chasing you—that's chasing us all.

Now all you have to do is go out there and make the right choices day after day, one day at a time.

INDEX

Dr. Howard M. Shapiro

Dr. Howard M. Shapiro changed the way America lost weight with his *New York Times* bestseller *Picture Perfect Weight Loss.* He is the founder and director of Howard M. Shapiro Medical Associates, a private multidisciplinary medical office in New York City that specializes in weight control, nutrition counseling and life management. He has been featured in the *New York Times, USA TODAY* and *Vogue,* among others, and has been a frequent guest on numerous national television and radio programs, including *Oprah, Today, Good Morning America* and *The View.* Dr. Shapiro worked extensively with the New York Police Department and the Fire Department of New York, helping them lose a total of 2,544 pounds. Visit his Web site at www.drhowardshapiro.com.

Franklin Becker

Franklin Becker has served as executive chef at several of New York's premier restaurants and his work has been featured in the *New York Times, New York* magazine, *Esquire* and *People.* At the age of twenty-seven, he was diagnosed with type 2 diabetes. Following his diagnosis, Chef Becker lost 35 pounds and transformed his cooking style to create dazzling dishes that are healthy and flavorful. Chef Becker currently presides over Abe & Arthur's restaurant, located in New York City's Meatpacking district. Visit his Web site at www.cheffranklinbecker.com.